PN Maternal Newborn Nursing
REVIEW MODULE EDITION 10.0

Contributors

Norma Jean E. Henry, MSN/Ed, RN

Honey C. Holman, MSN, RN

Kellie Wilford, MSN, RN

Marsha S. Barlow, MSN, RN

Mendy G. McMichael, DNP, MSN, RN

Consultants

Christi Blair, MSN, RN

Maureen D. Abraham, RNC, MSN, CNE

INTELLECTUAL PROPERTY NOTICE

Director of content review: Kristen Lawler

Director of development: Derek Prater

Project management: Nicole Burke

Coordination of content review: Norma Jean E. Henry, Honey C. Holman

Copy editing: Kelly Von Lunen, Bethany Phillips

Layout: Spring Lenox, Randi Hardy, Charves Hervey, Rachel Cohen

Illustrations: Randi Hardy

Online media: Morgan Smith, Ron Hanson, Nicole Lobdell, Brant Stacy

Cover design: Jason Buck

Interior book design: Spring Lenox

IMPORTANT NOTICE TO THE READER

User's Guide

Welcome to the Assessment Technologies Institute® PN Maternal Newborn Nursing Review Module Edition 10.0. The mission of ATI's Content Mastery Series® Review Modules is to provide user-friendly compendiums of nursing knowledge that will:

- Help you locate important information quickly.
- Assist in your learning efforts.
- Provide exercises for applying your nursing knowledge.
- Facilitate your entry into the nursing profession as a newly licensed nurse.

This newest edition of the Review Modules has been redesigned to optimize your learning experience. We've fit more content into less space and have done so in a way that will make it even easier for you to find and understand the information you need.

ORGANIZATION

This Review Module is organized into units covering antepartum, intrapartum, postpartum, and newborn nursing care. Chapters within these units conform to one of three organizing principles for presenting the content.

- Nursing concepts
- Procedures
- Complications of pregnancy

Nursing concepts chapters begin with an overview describing the central concept and its relevance to nursing. Subordinate themes are covered in outline form to demonstrate relationships and present the information in a clear, succinct manner.

Procedures chapters include an overview describing the procedure(s) covered in the chapter. These chapters provide nursing knowledge relevant to each procedure, including indications, nursing considerations, and complications.

Complications of pregnancy chapters include an overview describing the complication; assessment, including risk factors and expected findings; and patient-centered care, including nursing care, medications, and client education.

ACTIVE LEARNING SCENARIOS AND APPLICATION EXERCISES

Each chapter includes opportunities for you to test your knowledge and to practice applying that knowledge. Active Learning Scenario exercises pose a nursing scenario and then direct you to use an ATI Active Learning Template (included at the back of this book) to record the important knowledge a nurse should apply to the scenario. An example is then provided to which you can compare your completed Active Learning Template. The Application Exercises include NCLEX-style questions, such as multiple-choice and multiple-select items, providing you with opportunities to practice answering the kinds of questions you might expect to see on ATI assessments or the NCLEX. After the Application Exercises, an answer key is provided, along with rationales.

NCLEX® CONNECTIONS

To prepare for the NCLEX-PN, it is important to understand how the content in this Review Module is connected to the NCLEX-PN test plan. You can find information on the detailed test plan at the National Council of State Boards of Nursing's website, www.ncsbn.org. When reviewing content in this Review Module, regularly ask yourself, "How does this content fit into the test plan, and what types of questions related to this content should I expect?"

To help you in this process, we've included NCLEX Connections at the beginning of each unit and with each question in the Application Exercises Answer Keys. The NCLEX Connections at the beginning of each unit point out areas of the detailed test plan that relate to the content within that unit. The NCLEX Connections attached to the Application Exercises Answer Keys demonstrate how each exercise fits within the detailed content outline. These NCLEX Connections will help you understand how the detailed content outline is organized, starting with major client needs categories and subcategories and followed by related content areas and tasks. The major client needs categories are:

- Safe and Effective Care Environment
  - Management of Care
  - Safety and Infection Control
- Health Promotion and Maintenance
- Psychosocial Integrity
- Physiological Integrity
  - Basic Care and Comfort
  - Pharmacological and Parenteral Therapies
  - Reduction of Risk Potential
  - Physiological Adaptation

An NCLEX Connection might, for example, alert you that content within a unit is related to:

- Health Promotion and Maintenance
  - Ante/Intra/Postpartum and Newborn Care
    - Assess client psychosocial response to pregnancy.

QSEN COMPETENCIES

As you use the Review Modules, you will note the integration of the Quality and Safety Education for Nurses (QSEN) competencies throughout the chapters. These competencies are integral components of the curriculum of many nursing programs in the United States and prepare you to provide safe, high-quality care as a newly licensed nurse. Icons appear to draw your attention to the six QSEN competencies.

Safety: The minimization of risk factors that could cause injury or harm while promoting quality care and maintaining a secure environment for clients, self, and others.

Patient-Centered Care: The provision of caring and compassionate, culturally sensitive care that addresses clients' physiological, psychological, sociological, spiritual, and cultural needs, preferences, and values.

Evidence-Based Practice: The use of current knowledge from research and other credible sources, on which to base clinical judgment and client care.

Informatics: The use of information technology as a communication and information-gathering tool that supports clinical decision-making and scientifically based nursing practice.

Quality Improvement: Care related and organizational processes that involve the development and implementation of a plan to improve health care services and better meet clients' needs.

Teamwork and Collaboration: The delivery of client care in partnership with multidisciplinary members of the health care team to achieve continuity of care and positive client outcomes.

ICONS

Icons are used throughout the Review Module to draw your attention to particular areas. Keep an eye out for these icons.

(N) This icon is used for NCLEX Connections.

(G) This icon indicates gerontological considerations, or knowledge specific to the care of older adult clients.

Qs This icon is used for content related to safety and is a QSEN competency. When you see this icon, take note of safety concerns or steps that nurses can take to ensure client safety and a safe environment.

Qpcc This icon is a QSEN competency that indicates the importance of a holistic approach to providing care.

Qebp This icon, a QSEN competency, points out the integration of research into clinical practice.

Qi This icon is a QSEN competency and highlights the use of information technology to support nursing practice.

Qqi This icon is used to focus on the QSEN competency of integrating planning processes to meet clients' needs.

Qtc This icon highlights the QSEN competency of care delivery using an interprofessional approach.

M◇ This icon appears at the top-right of pages and indicates availability of an online media supplement, such as a graphic, animation, or video. If you have an electronic copy of the Review Module, this icon will appear alongside clickable links to media supplements. If you have a hard copy version of the Review Module, visit www.atitesting.com for details on how to access these features.

FEEDBACK

ATI welcomes feedback regarding this Review Module. Please provide comments to comments@atitesting.com.

Table of Contents

NCLEX® Connections

When reviewing the following chapters, keep in mind the relevant topics and tasks of the NCLEX outline, in particular:

Health Promotion and Maintenance

ANTE/INTRA/POSTPARTUM AND NEWBORN CARE: Assist in performing client nonstress test.

DATA COLLECTION TECHNIQUES: Collect data for health history (client medical history, family medical history).

HEALTH PROMOTION/DISEASE PREVENTION: Identify clients in need of immunizations (required and voluntary).

HIGH-RISK BEHAVIORS: Provide information for prevention of high-risk behaviors.

LIFESTYLE CHOICES: Recognize the client's need/desire for contraception.

Basic Care and Comfort

NONPHARMACOLOGICAL COMFORT INTERVENTIONS: Use alternative/complementary therapy in providing client care (such as music therapy).

NUTRITION AND ORAL HYDRATION: Monitor and provide for nutritional needs of clients.

Pharmacological Therapies

ADVERSE EFFECTS/CONTRAINDICATIONS/SIDE EFFECTS/ INTERACTIONS: Reinforce client teaching on possible effects of medications (common side effects or adverse effects, when to notify primary health care provider).

EXPECTED ACTIONS/OUTCOMES: Identify client expected response to medication.

MEDICATION ADMINISTRATION: Identify client need for PRN medications.

Reduction of Risk Potential

DIAGNOSTIC TESTS: Reinforce client teaching about diagnostic tests.

LABORATORY VALUES: Monitor diagnostic or laboratory test results.

POTENTIAL FOR ALTERATIONS IN BODY SYSTEMS: Identify signs or symptoms of potential prenatal complications.

Physiological Adaptation

ALTERATIONS IN BODY SYSTEMS: Provide care for a client experiencing complications of pregnancy/labor and/or delivery (eclampsia, precipitous labor, hemorrhage).

CHAPTER 1 Contraception

Contraception refers to strategies or devices used to reduce the risk of fertilization or implantation in an attempt to prevent pregnancy. The human ovum can be fertilized no later than 24 hr after ovulation. Motile sperm have been recovered from the uterus and oviducts as long as 60 hr after coitus, but their ability to fertilize the ovum probably lasts no longer than 48 hr.

The nurse should collect data related to the clients' need, desire, and preferences for contraception. The nurse should identify contraindications and provide support of the client's chosen contraceptive method. Qpcc

Sexual partners often make a joint decision regarding a desired preference (vasectomy, tubal ligation). During the postpartum time, the nurse should identify and discuss the client's future contraceptive plans.

Expected outcomes for family planning methods include preventing pregnancy until a desired time. Nurses should support clients in making the decision that is best for their individual situations.

Methods of contraception include natural family planning; barrier, hormonal, and intrauterine methods; and surgical procedures.

NATURAL FAMILY PLANNING (FERTILITY AWARENESS-BASED METHODS)

Abstinence

Abstaining from sexual intercourse eliminates the possibility of sperm entering the vagina.

CLIENT EDUCATION: Refrain from sexual intercourse. This method can be associated with saying "no," but it also can incorporate other gratifying sexual activities (affectionate touching, communication, holding hands, kissing, massage, oral and manual stimulation).

ADVANTAGES
- Most effective method of birth control.
- Clients can use abstinence during fertile periods (rhythm method), but it requires an understanding of the menstrual cycle and fertility awareness.
- There is no risk of sexually transmitted infections (STIs) if there is no genital contact.

DISADVANTAGES: Requires self-control

RISKS: If complete abstinence is maintained, there are no risks.

Coitus interruptus (withdrawal)

Withdrawal of penis from vagina prior to ejaculation.

CLIENT EDUCATION: Be aware of fluids leaking from the penis.

ADVANTAGES: Possible choice for monogamous couples who do not have another contraceptives available.

DISADVANTAGES
- One of the least effective methods of contraception.
- No protection against STIs.

RISKS
- Influenced by male partner's control.
- Leakage of fluid that contains spermatozoa prior to ejaculation can be deposited in vagina.
- Risk of pregnancy.

Calendar method

A woman records her menstrual cycle by calculating her fertile period based on the assumption that ovulation occurs about 14 days before the onset of her next menstrual cycle, and avoids intercourse during that period. Also taken into account is the timing of intercourse with this method, because sperm are viable for 48 to 72 hr, and the ovum is viable for about 24 hr.

CLIENT EDUCATION

- Accurately record the number of days in each cycle counting from the first day of menses for at least six cycles.
- The start of the fertile period is figured by subtracting 18 days from the number of days in the woman's shortest cycle.
- The end of the fertile period is established by subtracting 11 days from the number of days of the longest cycle.

> **FOR EXAMPLE**
> Shortest cycle: 26 − 18 = 8th day
> Longest cycle: 30 − 11 = 19th day
> Fertile period is days 8 through 19.
> Refrain from intercourse during these days to avoid conception.

ADVANTAGES

- Most useful when combined with basal body temperature or cervical mucus method
- Inexpensive

DISADVANTAGES

- Not a very reliable technique
- Does not protect against STIs
- Requires accurate record-keeping
- Requires compliance regarding abstinence during fertile periods

RISKS

- Various factors can affect and change the time of ovulation and cause unpredictable menstrual cycles.
- Risk of pregnancy.

Basal body temperature

Temperature can drop slightly at the time of ovulation. This can be used to facilitate conception, or be used as a natural contraceptive.

CLIENT EDUCATION: Measure oral temperature prior to getting out of bed each morning to monitor ovulation.

ADVANTAGES: Inexpensive, convenient, and no adverse effects

DISADVANTAGES

- Reliability is influenced by many variables that can cause inaccurate interpretation of temperature changes (stress, fatigue, illness, alcohol, warmth of sleeping environment).
- Does not protect against STIs.

RISKS: Risk of pregnancy

Symptom-based method (cervical mucus)

Fertility awareness method based on ovulation. Ovulation occurs approximately 14 days prior to the next menstrual cycle, which is when a woman is fertile. Following ovulation, the cervical mucus becomes thin and flexible under the influence of estrogen and progesterone to allow for sperm viability and motility. The ability for the mucus to stretch between the fingers is greatest during ovulation. This is referred to as spinnbarkeit sign.

CLIENT EDUCATION

- Engage in good hand hygiene prior to and following assessment.
- Begin examining mucus from the last day of the menstrual cycle.
- Mucus is obtained from the vaginal introitus. It is not necessary to reach into the vagina to the cervix.
- Do not douche prior to assessment.

ADVANTAGES

- A woman can become knowledgeable in recognizing her own mucus characteristics at ovulation, and self-evaluation can be very accurate.
- Self-evaluation of cervical mucus can be diagnostically helpful in determining the start of ovulation while breastfeeding, noting the commencement of menopause, and planning a desired pregnancy.

DISADVANTAGES

- Some women are uncomfortable with touching their genitals and mucus, and therefore find this method objectionable.
- Does not protect against STIs.

RISKS/POSSIBLE COMPLICATIONS

- Assessment of cervical mucus characteristics can be inaccurate if mucus is mixed with semen, blood, contraceptive foams, or discharge from infections.
- Risk of pregnancy.

BARRIER METHODS

Male condom

A thin rubber sheath worn on the penis during sexual intercourse as a contraceptive or as protection against infection. Male condoms can be made of latex rubber, polyurethane, or natural membrane.

CLIENT EDUCATION

- Place a condom on the erect penis, leaving an empty space at the tip for a sperm reservoir.
- Following ejaculation, withdraw the penis from the vagina while holding the rim of the condom to prevent any semen spillage to the vulva or vaginal area.
- Can be used in conjunction with spermicidal gel or cream to increase effectiveness.

ADVANTAGES

- Protects against STIs and involves the male in the birth control method
- No adverse effects
- Readily accessible

DISADVANTAGES

- High rate of noncompliance.
- Can reduce spontaneity of intercourse.
- The penis must be erect to apply a condom.
- Withdrawing the penis while still erect can interfere with sexual intercourse.

RISKS/COMPLICATIONS/CONTRAINDICATIONS

- Condoms can rupture or leak, potentially resulting in pregnancy.
- Condoms have a one-time usage, which creates a replacement cost.
- Condoms made of latex should not be worn by those who are sensitive or allergic to latex.
- Only water-soluble lubricants should be used with latex condoms to avoid condom breakage.

Female condom

Vaginal sheath made of nitrile, a nonlatex synthetic rubber with flexible rings on both ends

CLIENT EDUCATION: The closed end of the pouch is inserted into the vagina by the client prior to intercourse and anchored around the cervix. The open ring covers the labia. The condom is removed and thrown away after intercourse.

ADVANTAGES: Offers protection against pregnancy and STIs

Diaphragm and spermicide

A dome-shaped cup with a flexible rim made of silicone that fits snugly over the cervix with spermicidal cream or gel placed into the dome and around the rim. Diaphragms are available in different sizes.

CLIENT EDUCATION

- Be properly fitted with a diaphragm by a provider.
- Replace every 2 years and refit for a 20% weight fluctuation, after abdominal or pelvic surgery, and after every pregnancy.
- Requires proper insertion and removal. Prior to coitus, the diaphragm is inserted vaginally over the cervix with spermicidal jelly or cream that is applied to the cervical side of the dome and around the rim. The diaphragm can be inserted up to 6 hr before intercourse and must stay in place 6 hr after intercourse but for no more than 24 hr.
- Reapply spermicide with each act of coitus.
- Empty the bladder prior to insertion of the diaphragm.
- Wash the diaphragm with mild soap and warm water after each use.

ADVANTAGES: Gives a woman control over contraception

DISADVANTAGES

- Diaphragms are inconvenient; interfere with spontaneity; and require reapplication with spermicidal gel, cream, or foam with each act of coitus to be effective.
- Requires a prescription and a visit to a provider.
- Must be inserted correctly to be effective.
- Does not protect against STIs.

RISKS/COMPLICATIONS/CONTRAINDICATIONS

- Not recommended for clients who have a history of toxic shock syndrome (TSS), or frequent, recurrent urinary tract infections.
- Increased risk of acquiring TSS, which is caused by a bacterial infection. Findings include high fever, a faint feeling, drop in blood pressure, watery diarrhea, headache, and muscle aches.
- Proper hand hygiene aids in prevention of TSS, as well as removing diaphragm promptly at 6 hr following coitus.
- Risk of allergic reaction

Cervical cap and spermicide

Silicone rubber cap that fits snugly around the base of the cervix. Cervical caps come in three sizes.

CLIENT EDUCATION

- Can be inserted up to 6 hr before intercourse and needs to be left in place at least 6 hr after intercourse but for no more than 48 hr at a time.
- Replace every 2 years and refit after any gynecological surgery, birth, or major weight fluctuation.
- Cervical cap should be washed with mild soap and warm water after each use.

DISADVANTAGES

- Possible risk of acquiring TSS
- Risk of allergic reaction
- Does not protect against STIs

RISKS/COMPLICATIONS/CONTRAINDICATIONS: Not for women who have abnormal Pap test results or those who have a history of TSS

Contraceptive sponge

Small, round, polyurethane sponge containing spermicide

CLIENT EDUCATION

- It is designed to fit over the cervix, and is one size fits all.
- Should be left in place for 6 hr after intercourse and provides protection for up to 24 hr.

DISADVANTAGES: Does not protect against STIs

HORMONAL METHODS

Combined oral contraceptives

Hormonal contraception containing estrogen and progestin, which acts by suppressing ovulation, thickening the cervical mucus to block semen, and altering the uterine decidua to prevent implantation

CLIENT EDUCATION
- Medication requires a prescription and follow-up appointments with the provider.
- Medication requires consistent and proper use to be effective.
- Observe for adverse effects and danger indications of medication. Indicators include chest pain, shortness of breath, leg pain from a possible clot, headache, eye problems from a stroke, and hypertension.
- In the event of missing a dose, if one pill is missed, take one as soon as possible; if two or three pills are missed, follow the manufacturer's instructions. Use alternative forms of contraception or abstinence to prevent pregnancy until regular dosing is resumed.

ADVANTAGES
- Highly effective if taken correctly and consistently
- Noncontraceptive benefits of combined hormonal contraception containing low-dose estrogen (less than 35 mcg)
  - Decreased menstrual blood loss
  - Decreased iron deficiency anemia
  - Regulation of menorrhagia and irregular cycles
  - Reduced incidence of dysmenorrhea and premenstrual manifestations
- Offers protection against endometrial, ovarian, and colon cancer, reduces the incidence of benign breast disease, improves acne, and protects against the development of functional ovarian cysts

DISADVANTAGES
- Do not protect against STIs.
- Can increase the risk of thromboembolism, stroke, heart attack, hypertension, gallbladder disease, liver tumor.
- Exacerbates conditions affected by fluid retention (migraine, epilepsy, asthma, kidney, heart disease).
- Adverse effects include headache, nausea, breast tenderness, and breakthrough bleeding.
  - Common adverse effects of estrogen component include nausea, breast tenderness, and fluid retention.
  - Common adverse effects of progestin component include increased appetite, tiredness, depression, breast tenderness, oily skin and scalp, and hirsutism.

RISKS/COMPLICATIONS/CONTRAINDICATIONS
- Women who have a history of thromboembolic disorders, stroke, heart attack, coronary artery disease, gallbladder disease, cirrhosis or liver tumor, headache with focal neurological manifestations, uncontrolled hypertension, diabetes mellitus with vascular involvement, breast or estrogen-related cancers, pregnancy, lactating, less than 6 weeks postpartum, or smoking (if older than 35 years) are advised not to take oral contraceptive medications.
- Oral contraceptive effectiveness decreases when taking medications that affect liver enzymes, such as anticonvulsants and some antibiotics.

Progestin-only pills (minipill)

Oral progestins that provide the same action as combined oral contraceptives

CLIENT EDUCATION
- Take the pill at the same time daily to ensure effectiveness secondary to a low dose of progestin.
- Do not miss a pill.
- Another form of birth control might be needed during the first month of use to prevent pregnancy.

ADVANTAGES
- Fewer adverse effects when compared with a combined oral contraceptive
- Considered safe to take while breastfeeding

DISADVANTAGES
- Less effective in suppressing ovulation than combined oral contraceptives
- Increased occurrence of ovarian cysts
- No protection against STIs
- Adverse effects include breakthrough, irregular, vaginal bleeding (frequently reported/most common); headache; nausea; and breast tenderness.

RISKS/COMPLICATIONS/CONTRAINDICATIONS
- Oral contraceptive effectiveness decreases when taking medications that affect liver enzymes, such as anticonvulsants and some antibiotics.
- Contraindications include bariatric surgery, lupus, severe cirrhosis, liver tumors, and current or past breast cancer.

Emergency oral contraceptive

Morning-after pill that prevents fertilization

CLIENT EDUCATION
- Take pill within 72 hr after unprotected coitus.
- The provider might recommend an over-the-counter antiemetic 1 hr prior to each dose to counteract nausea that can occur with high doses of estrogen and progestin.
- Have an evaluation for pregnancy if menstruation does not begin within 21 days.
- Provide reinforcement of teaching about contraception and modification of sexual behaviors that are risky.
- Considered a form of emergency birth control.

ADVANTAGES
- Not taken on a regular basis.
- Anyone, regardless of age or gender, is allowed to purchase emergency oral contraceptive at a pharmacy.

DISADVANTAGES
- Nausea, heavier than normal menstrual bleeding, lower abdominal pain, fatigue, and headache.
- Does not provide long-term contraception.
- Does not terminate an established pregnancy.
- Does not protect against STIs.

RISKS/COMPLICATIONS/CONTRAINDICATIONS
- Contraindicated if a client is pregnant or has undiagnosed abnormal vaginal bleeding.
- If menstruation does not start within 1 week of expected date, a client might be pregnant.

Transdermal contraceptive patch

Contains norelgestromin (progesterone) and ethinyl estradiol, which is delivered at continuous levels through the skin into subcutaneous tissue

CLIENT EDUCATION
- Apply the patch to dry skin overlying subcutaneous tissue of the buttock, abdomen, upper arm, or torso, excluding breast area.
- Requires patch replacement once a week.
- Apply the patch the same day of the week for 3 weeks with no application on the fourth week.

ADVANTAGES
- Maintains consistent blood levels of hormone
- Avoids liver metabolism of medication because it is not absorbed in the gastrointestinal tract
- Decreases risk of forgetting daily pill

DISADVANTAGES
- Does not protect against STIs
- Same adverse effects as oral contraceptives. Risk of deep-vein thrombosis and venous thromboembolism can be slightly higher in women using the patch because the hormones get into the bloodstream and are processed by the body differently than hormones from OCPs.
- Skin reaction can occur from patch application.

RISKS/COMPLICATIONS/CONTRAINDICATIONS
- Same as those of oral contraceptives
- Avoid applying of patch to skin rashes or lesions.
- Less effective in women who weigh more than 198 lb.

Injectable progestins

Medroxyprogesterone is an intramuscular or subcutaneous injection given to a female client every 11 to 13 weeks

CLIENT EDUCATION
- Start of injections should be during the first 5 days of a client's menstrual cycle and every 11 to 13 weeks thereafter. Injections in postpartum nonbreastfeeding women should begin within 5 days following delivery. For breastfeeding women, injections should start in the sixth week postpartum.
- Keep follow-up appointments.
- Maintain an adequate intake of calcium and vitamin D.

ADVANTAGES
- Very effective and requires only four injections per year
- Does not impair lactation
- Possible absence of periods and decrease in bleeding
- Decreased risk of uterine cancer if used long-term

DISADVANTAGES
- Adverse effects include decrease in bone mineral density, weight gain, increase in depression, and irregular vaginal spotting or bleeding.
- Does not protect against STIs.
- Return to fertility can be delayed up to 18 months after discontinuation.
- The client should only use as a long-term method of birth control (more than 2 years) if other birth control methods are inadequate.

RISKS/COMPLICATIONS/CONTRAINDICATIONS
- Avoid massaging injection site following administration to avoid accelerating medication absorption, which will shorten the duration of its effectiveness.
- Contraindications include breast cancer, evidence of current cardiovascular disease, abnormal liver function, liver tumors, and unexplained vaginal bleeding.

Contraceptive vaginal ring

Contains etonogestrel and ethinyl estradiol that is delivered at continuous levels vaginally

CLIENT EDUCATION
- Insert the ring vaginally.
- Requires ring replacement after 3 weeks, and placement of new vaginal ring within 7 days. Insertion should occur on the same day of the week monthly.

ADVANTAGES
- Does not have to be fitted
- Decreases the risk of forgetting to take the pill
- Vaginal route of delivery increases bioavailability of hormones, enabling lower dose and reducing adverse effects.

DISADVANTAGES
- Does not protect against STIs.
- Same adverse effects as oral contraceptives.
- Some clients report discomfort during intercourse. The ring can be removed for up to 3 hr without compromising effectiveness.

RISKS/COMPLICATIONS/CONTRAINDICATIONS
- Blood clots, hypertension, stroke, heart attack
- Vaginal irritation, increased vaginal secretions, headache, weight gain, nausea

Implantable progestin

Requires a minor surgical procedure to subdermally implant and remove a single rod containing etonogestrel on the inner side of the upper aspect of the arm

CLIENT EDUCATION: Avoid trauma to the area of implantation.

ADVANTAGES
- Effective continuous contraception for 3 years
- Can be inserted immediately after elective abortion, miscarriage, childbirth, and while breastfeeding
- Reversible
- Can be used by mothers who are breastfeeding after 4 weeks postpartum

DISADVANTAGES
- Etonogestrel can cause irregular menstrual bleeding.
- Does not protect against STIs.
- Adverse effects include irregular and unpredictable menstruation (most common), mood changes, headache, acne, depression, decreased bone density, and weight gain.

RISKS/COMPLICATIONS/CONTRAINDICATIONS
- Increased risk of ectopic pregnancy if pregnancy occurs.
- Contraindications include unexplained vaginal bleeding, lupus, severe cirrhosis, liver tumors, and breast cancer.

Intrauterine device (IUD)

A chemically active T-shaped device that is inserted through the cervix and placed in the uterus by the provider. Releases a chemical substance that damages sperm in transit to the uterine tubes and prevents fertilization. The most effective contraceptive methods at preventing pregnancy are the long-acting reversible contraceptive (LARC) methods: implant and IUDs. IUDs can be used by nulliparous and multiparous women.

CLIENT EDUCATION

- Monitor the device monthly after menstruation to ensure the presence of the small string that hangs from the device into the upper part of the vagina to rule out migration or expulsion of the device.
- Report to the provider late or abnormal spotting or bleeding, abdominal pain or pain with intercourse, abnormal or foul-smelling vaginal discharge, fever, chills, a change in string length, or if IUD cannot be located.

ADVANTAGES

- An IUD can maintain effectiveness for 1 to 10 years (hormonal: 3 to 5 years; copper: 10 years).
- Can be inserted immediately after elective abortion, miscarriage, childbirth, and while breastfeeding
- Contraception can be reversed with immediate return to fertility.
- Does not interfere with spontaneity
- Safe for mothers who are breastfeeding
- 99% effective in preventing pregnancy
- Hormonal IUDs: decreased menstrual pain and heavy bleeding
- Copper IUD: no hormones, so safe for women cautioned against hormonal birth control methods

DISADVANTAGES

- Can increase the risk of pelvic inflammatory disease, uterine perforation, or ectopic pregnancy
- Can be expelled
- Does not protect from STIs
- Hormonal IUD: spotting, irregular bleeding, headache, nausea, depression, breast tenderness
- Copper IUD: increase in menstrual pain and bleeding

RISKS/CONTRAINDICATIONS

- Recommended for clients in a monogamous relationship due to the risks of STIs
- Can cause irregular menstrual bleeding
- Risk of bacterial vaginosis, uterine perforation, or uterine expulsion
- Must be removed in the event of pregnancy

CONTRAINDICATIONS: Active pelvic infection, abnormal uterine bleeding, severe uterine distortion; for copper IUD also Wilson's disease and copper allergy

TRANSCERVICAL STERILIZATION

- Insertion of small flexible agents through the vagina and cervix into the fallopian tubes. This results in the development of scar tissue in the tubes preventing conception.
- Examination is done after 3 months to ensure fallopian tubes are blocked.

CLIENT EDUCATION: Most clients can resume normal activities within 1 day of the procedure.

ADVANTAGES

- Quick procedure that requires no general anesthesia
- Nonhormonal means of birth control
- 99.8% effective in preventing pregnancy
- Rapid return to normal activities of daily living

DISADVANTAGES

- Not reversible
- Not intended for use in the client who is postpartum
- Delay in effectiveness for 3 months. The client should use an alternative means of birth control until confirmation of blocked fallopian tubes occurs.
- Changes in menstrual patterns
- Does not protect against STIs

RISKS/COMPLICATIONS/CONTRAINDICATIONS

- Perforation can occur.
- Unwanted pregnancy can occur if a client has unprotected sexual intercourse during the first 3 months following the procedure.
- Increased risk of ectopic pregnancy if pregnancy occurs.

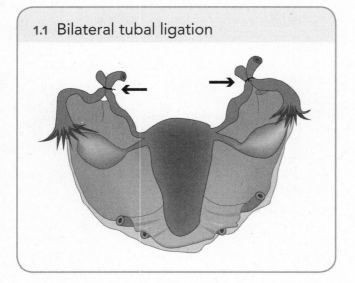

1.1 Bilateral tubal ligation

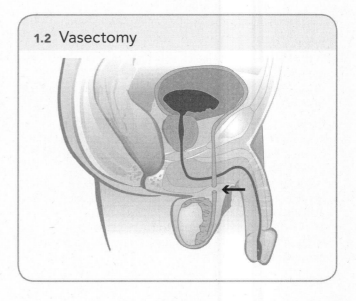

1.2 Vasectomy

SURGICAL METHODS

Female sterilization (bilateral tubal ligation)

A surgical procedure consisting of severance and/or burning or blocking the fallopian tubes to prevent fertilization (1.1)

PROCEDURE: Cutting, burning, or blocking of the fallopian tubes to prevent the ovum from being fertilized by the sperm.

ADVANTAGES
- Permanent contraception
- Can be done immediately after childbirth within 24 to 48 hr
- Sexual function is unaffected.

DISADVANTAGES
- A surgical procedure carrying risks related to anesthesia, complications, infection, hemorrhage, or trauma
- Considered irreversible in the event that a client desires conception
- Does not protect against STIs

RISKS: Risk of ectopic pregnancy if pregnancy occurs

Male sterilization (vasectomy)

A surgical procedure consisting of ligation and severance of the vas deferens. (1.2)

PROCEDURE: Cutting of the vas deferens in the male as a form of permanent sterilization. Sterility is delayed until the proximal portion of the vas deferens is cleared of all remaining sperm (approximately 20 ejaculations).

CLIENT EDUCATION
- Use alternate forms of birth control for approximately 20 ejaculations or 1 week to several months to allow all of the sperm to clear the vas deferens. This will ensure complete male infertility.
- Following the procedure, scrotal support and moderate activity for a couple of days is recommended to reduce discomfort.
- Follow-up is important for sperm count.

ADVANTAGES
- Permanent contraceptive method.
- Procedure is short, safe, and simple.
- Sexual function is not impaired.

DISADVANTAGES
- Requires surgery.
- Reversal is possible but not always successful.
- Does not protect against STIs.

COMPLICATIONS: Rare, but can include bleeding, infection, and anesthesia reaction

Application Exercises

1. A nurse in a health clinic is reviewing contraceptive use with a group of adolescent clients. Which of the following statements by an adolescent reflects an understanding of the teaching?

   A. "A water-soluble lubricant should be used with condoms."

   B. "A diaphragm should be removed 2 hours after intercourse."

   C. "Oral contraceptives can worsen a case of acne."

   D. "A contraceptive patch is replaced once a month."

2. A nurse is reinforcing teaching with a client who is taking an oral contraceptive about danger indications to report to her provider. The nurse determines the client understands the teaching when the client states the need to report which of the following manifestations?

   A. Reduced menstrual flow

   B. Breast tenderness

   C. Shortness of breath

   D. Headaches

3. A nurse in an obstetrical clinic is reinforcing teaching with a client about using an IUD for contraception. Which of the following statements by the client indicates an understanding of the information?

   A. "An IUD should be replaced annually during a pelvic exam."

   B. "I cannot get an IUD until after I've had a child."

   C. "I should expect intermittent abdominal pain while the IUD is in place."

   D. "A change in the string length of my IUD is expected."

4. A nurse is reinforcing teaching with a client about potential adverse effects of implantable progestins. Which of the following adverse effects should the nurse include? (Select all that apply.)

   A. Tinnitus

   B. Irregular vaginal bleeding

   C. Weight gain

   D. Breast changes

   E. Gingival hyperplasia

5. A nurse in a clinic is reinforcing teaching with a client about her new prescription for medroxyprogesterone. Which of the following information should the nurse include? (Select all that apply.)

   A. "Weight loss can occur."

   B. "You are protected against STIs."

   C. "You should increase your intake of calcium."

   D. "You should avoid taking antibiotics."

   E. "Irregular vaginal spotting can occur."

SURGICAL METHODS

Female sterilization (bilateral tubal ligation)

A surgical procedure consisting of severance and/or burning or blocking the fallopian tubes to prevent fertilization (1.1)

PROCEDURE: Cutting, burning, or blocking of the fallopian tubes to prevent the ovum from being fertilized by the sperm.

ADVANTAGES
- Permanent contraception
- Can be done immediately after childbirth within 24 to 48 hr
- Sexual function is unaffected.

DISADVANTAGES
- A surgical procedure carrying risks related to anesthesia, complications, infection, hemorrhage, or trauma
- Considered irreversible in the event that a client desires conception
- Does not protect against STIs

RISKS: Risk of ectopic pregnancy if pregnancy occurs

Male sterilization (vasectomy)

A surgical procedure consisting of ligation and severance of the vas deferens. (1.2)

PROCEDURE: Cutting of the vas deferens in the male as a form of permanent sterilization. Sterility is delayed until the proximal portion of the vas deferens is cleared of all remaining sperm (approximately 20 ejaculations).

CLIENT EDUCATION
- Use alternate forms of birth control for approximately 20 ejaculations or 1 week to several months to allow all of the sperm to clear the vas deferens. This will ensure complete male infertility.
- Following the procedure, scrotal support and moderate activity for a couple of days is recommended to reduce discomfort.
- Follow-up is important for sperm count.

ADVANTAGES
- Permanent contraceptive method.
- Procedure is short, safe, and simple.
- Sexual function is not impaired.

DISADVANTAGES
- Requires surgery.
- Reversal is possible but not always successful.
- Does not protect against STIs.

COMPLICATIONS: Rare, but can include bleeding, infection, and anesthesia reaction

Application Exercises

1. A nurse in a health clinic is reviewing contraceptive use with a group of adolescent clients. Which of the following statements by an adolescent reflects an understanding of the teaching?

   A. "A water-soluble lubricant should be used with condoms."

   B. "A diaphragm should be removed 2 hours after intercourse."

   C. "Oral contraceptives can worsen a case of acne."

   D. "A contraceptive patch is replaced once a month."

2. A nurse is reinforcing teaching with a client who is taking an oral contraceptive about danger indications to report to her provider. The nurse determines the client understands the teaching when the client states the need to report which of the following manifestations?

   A. Reduced menstrual flow

   B. Breast tenderness

   C. Shortness of breath

   D. Headaches

3. A nurse in an obstetrical clinic is reinforcing teaching with a client about using an IUD for contraception. Which of the following statements by the client indicates an understanding of the information?

   A. "An IUD should be replaced annually during a pelvic exam."

   B. "I cannot get an IUD until after I've had a child."

   C. "I should plan on regaining fertility 5 months after the IUD is removed."

   D. "I will check to be sure the strings of the IUD are still present after my periods."

4. A nurse is reinforcing teaching with a client about potential adverse effects of implantable progestins. Which of the following adverse effects should the nurse include? (Select all that apply.)

   A. Tinnitus

   B. Irregular vaginal bleeding

   C. Weight gain

   D. Breast changes

   E. Gingival hyperplasia

5. A nurse in a clinic is reinforcing teaching with a client about her new prescription for medroxyprogesterone. Which of the following information should the nurse include? (Select all that apply.)

   A. "Weight loss can occur."

   B. "You are protected against STIs."

   C. "You should increase your intake of calcium."

   D. "You should avoid taking antibiotics."

   E. "Irregular vaginal spotting can occur."

Application Exercises Key

1. A. **CORRECT:** Condoms are used with water-soluble lubricants.

   B. A diaphragm should be removed no sooner than 6 hr and no later than 24 hr after intercourse.

   C. Acne is reduced when taking oral contraceptives.

   D. Contraceptive patches are replaced once a week.

   (N) NCLEX® Connection: Health Promotion and Maintenance, Lifestyle Choices

2. A. Reduced menstrual flow is a common adverse effect of oral contraceptives and usually subsides after a few months of use.

   B. Breast tenderness is a common adverse effect of oral contraceptives and usually subsides after a few months of use.

   C. **CORRECT:** The client should immediately report shortness of breath to the provider. This manifestation can indicate a pulmonary embolus or myocardial infarction.

   D. Headaches are a common adverse effect of oral contraceptives and usually subside after a few months of use.

   (N) NCLEX® Connection: Health Promotion and Maintenance, Lifestyle Choices

3. A. An IUD is replaced every 3 to 5 years, depending on the type of IUD used.

   B. Clients do not have to have given birth prior to the insertion of an IUD. It will be necessary for the client to have a negative pregnancy test prior to insertion of the IUD.

   C. Fertility will resume immediately following removal of the IUD.

   D. **CORRECT:** The client should check for presence of IUD strings following each menstruation to ensure the device is still present. A change in the length of the strings should be reported to the provider.

   (N) NCLEX® Connection: Health Promotion and Maintenance, Lifestyle Choices

4. A. Tinnitus is not an adverse effect of implantable progestins.

   B. **CORRECT:** Irregular vaginal bleeding is a potential adverse effect of implantable progestins.

   C. **CORRECT:** Weight gain is a potential adverse effect of implantable progestins.

   D. **CORRECT:** Breast changes are a potential adverse effect of implantable progestins.

   E. Gingival hyperplasia is not an adverse effect of implantable progestins.

   (N) NCLEX® Connection: Pharmacological Therapies, Adverse Effects/Contraindications/Side Effects/Interactions

5. A. Weight gain can occur when taking medroxyprogesterone.

   B. Medroxyprogesterone does not provide protection against STIs.

   C. **CORRECT:** Clients should take calcium and vitamin D to prevent loss of bone density, which can occur when taking medroxyprogesterone.

   D. Antibiotics are not contraindicated when taking medroxyprogesterone.

   E. **CORRECT:** Medroxyprogesterone can cause irregular vaginal bleeding.

   (N) NCLEX® Connection: Pharmacological Therapies, Adverse Effects/Contraindications/Side Effects/Interactions

PRACTICE Active Learning Scenario

A nurse is reinforcing teaching with a client who is considering a vasectomy. What information should the nurse include?

Use the ATI Active Learning Template: Therapeutic Procedure to complete this item.

DESCRIPTION OF PROCEDURE: Define the procedure.

INDICATIONS: Describe at least one advantage and one disadvantage of this form of contraception.

CLIENT EDUCATION: Describe two client education points to reinforce.

PRACTICE Answer

Using the ATI Active Learning: Therapeutic Procedure

DESCRIPTION OF PROCEDURE: Surgical procedure involving ligation and severance of the vas deferens

INDICATIONS
- Advantages
  - Permanent contraceptive method
  - Procedure is short, safe, and simple
  - Sexual function is not impaired
- Disadvantages
  - A surgical procedure
  - Considered irreversible

CLIENT EDUCATION
- Scrotal support and moderate activity are recommended for several days after the procedure to improve comfort.
- Use an alternate form of contraception for approximately 20 ejaculations to ensure that the vas deferens is cleared of remaining sperm.
- Have a follow-up sperm count.

(N) NCLEX® Connection: Reduction of Risk Potential, Potential for Complications of Diagnostic Tests/Treatments/Procedures

CALCULATING DELIVERY DATE AND NUMBER OF PREGNANCIES

Nägele's rule: Take the first day of the client's last menstrual cycle, subtract 3 months, and then add 7 days and 1 year, adjusting for the year as necessary.

Measurement of fundal height in centimeters from the symphysis pubis to the top of the uterine fundus (between 18 and 30 weeks of gestation) approximates the gestational age

Gravidity: number of pregnancies
- Nulligravida: a client who has never been pregnant
- Primigravida: a client in her first pregnancy
- Multigravida: a client who has had two or more pregnancies

Parity: number of pregnancies in which the fetuses reach 20 weeks of pregnancy (not the total number of fetuses). Parity is not affected whether the fetus is born stillborn or alive.
- Nullipara: no pregnancy beyond the stage of viability
- Primipara: has completed one pregnancy to stage of viability
- Multipara: has completed two or more pregnancies to stage of viability

Viability: The point when an fetus has the capacity to survive outside the uterus. There is not a specific weeks of gestation. However, infants born between 22 to 25 weeks are considered on the threshold of viability.

GTPAL acronym
- Gravidity
- Term births (38 weeks or more)
- Preterm births (from viability up to 37 weeks)
- Abortions/miscarriages (prior to viability)
- Living children

PHYSIOLOGICAL STATUS OF PREGNANT CLIENTS

BODY SYSTEMS

Reproductive

Uterus increases in size and changes shape and position. Ovulation and menses cease during pregnancy.

Cardiovascular

Cardiac output increases (30% to 50%) and blood volume increases (30% to 45% at term) to meet the greater metabolic needs. Heart rate increases during pregnancy beginning around week 5 and reaches a peak (10 to 15/min above prepregnancy rate) around 32 weeks of pregnancy.

Respiratory

Maternal oxygen needs increase. During the last trimester, the size of the chest might enlarge, allowing for lung expansion as the uterus pushes upward. Respiratory rate increases and total lung capacity decreases.

Musculoskeletal

Body alterations and weight increase necessitate an adjustment in posture. Pelvic joints relax.

Gastrointestinal

Nausea and vomiting might occur due to hormonal changes or an increase of pressure within the abdominal cavity as the client's stomach and intestines are displaced within the abdomen. Constipation might occur due to increased transit time of food through the gastrointestinal tract and, thus, increased water absorption.

Renal

Filtration rate increases secondary to the influence of pregnancy hormones and an increase in blood volume and metabolic demands. The amount of urine produced remains the same. Urinary frequency is common during pregnancy.

Endocrine

The placenta becomes an endocrine organ that produces large amounts of hCG, progesterone, estrogen, human placental lactogen, and prostaglandins. Hormones are very active during pregnancy and function to maintain pregnancy and prepare the body for delivery.

BODY IMAGE CHANGES

- Due to physical and psychological changes that occur, the client requires support from the provider and family members.
- In the first trimester of pregnancy, physiological changes are not obvious. Many clients look forward to the changes so that the pregnancy will be more noticeable.
- During the second trimester, there are rapid physical changes due to the enlargement of the abdomen and breasts. These changes can affect a client's mobility. She might find herself losing her balance and feeling back or leg discomfort and fatigue. Skin changes also occur (stretch marks, hyperpigmentation). These factors can lead to a negative body image. The client might make statements of resentment toward the pregnancy and express anxiousness for the pregnancy to be over soon.

EXPECTED VITAL SIGNS

Blood pressure

- Blood pressure measurements are within the prepregnancy range during the first trimester. Q EBP
- **Systolic:** slight or no increase from prepregnancy levels
- **Diastolic:** slight decreases around 24 to 32 weeks; will gradually return to prepregnancy level by the end of the pregnancy
- The position of the client also might affect blood pressure.
  - In the supine position, blood pressure might appear to be lower due to the weight and pressure of the gravid uterus on the vena cava, which decreases venous blood flow to the heart.
  - Maternal hypotension and fetal hypoxia might occur, which is referred to as supine hypotensive syndrome or supine vena cava syndrome. Manifestations include dizziness, lightheadedness, and pale, clammy skin.
  - Encourage the client to lie on the left side, in a semi-Fowler's position, or, if supine, with a wedge placed under one hip to alleviate pressure to the vena cava.

Pulse

Pulse increases 10 to 15/min around 32 weeks of gestation and remains elevated throughout the remainder of the pregnancy.

Respirations

Respirations are unchanged or slightly increased. Respiratory changes in pregnancy are attributed to the elevation of the diaphragm by as much as 4 cm, as well as changes to the chest wall to facilitate increased maternal oxygen demands. Some shortness of breath might be noted.

EXPECTED FINDINGS

- The expected range for baseline fetal heart tones is 110 to 160/min. The presence of periodic accelerations in FHR are a positive indicator of an intact fetal CNS. Q EBP
- The client's heart changes in size and shape with resulting cardiac hypertrophy to accommodate increased blood volume and increased cardiac output. Heart sounds also change to accommodate the increase in blood volume with a more distinguishable splitting of S_1 and S_2, with S_3 more easily heard following 20 weeks of gestation. Murmurs also might be auscultated. Heart size and shape should return to normal shortly after delivery.
- Uterine size changes from a uterine weight of 50 to 1,000 g (0.1 to 2.2 lb). By 36 weeks of gestation, the top of the uterus and the fundus will reach the xiphoid process. This might cause the client to experience shortness of breath as the uterus pushes against the diaphragm.
- Cervical changes are obvious as a purplish-blue color extends into the vagina and labia, and the cervix becomes markedly soft.
- Breast changes occur due to hormones of pregnancy, with the breasts increasing in size and the areolae darkening.

SKIN CHANGES
- Chloasma: an increase of pigmentation on the face
- Linea nigra: dark line of pigmentation from the umbilicus extending to the pubic area
- Striae gravidarum: stretch marks most notably found on the abdomen and thighs

NURSING INTERVENTIONS

- Acknowledge the client's concerns about pregnancy and encourage sharing of these feelings while providing an atmosphere free of judgment.
- Discuss with the client the expected physiological changes and a possible timeline for a return to the prepregnant state.
- Refer the client to counseling if body image concerns appear to have a negative impact on the pregnancy.
- Reinforce education about the expected physiological and psychosocial changes. Common discomforts of pregnancy and ways to resolve those discomforts are reviewed during prenatal visits.
- The client is encouraged to keep all follow-up appointments and to contact the provider immediately if there is any bleeding, leakage of fluid, or contractions at any time during the pregnancy. Q s

Application Exercises

1. A nurse is caring for a client who is pregnant and states that her last menstrual period was April 1. Which of the following is the client's estimated date of delivery?

   A. January 8
   B. January 15
   C. February 8
   D. February 15

2. A nurse in a prenatal clinic is caring for a client who is in the first trimester of pregnancy. The client's health record includes this data: G3 T1 P0 A1 L1. How should the nurse interpret this information? (Select all that apply.)

   A. Client has delivered one newborn at term.
   B. Client has not experienced a preterm birth.
   C. Client has been through active labor.
   D. Client has had two prior pregnancies.
   E. Client has one living child.

3. A nurse is reviewing the health record of a client who is pregnant. The provider indicated the client exhibits probable signs of pregnancy. Which of the following findings should the nurse expect? (Select all that apply.)

   A. Enlarged Montgomery glands
   B. Goodell's sign
   C. Ballottement
   D. Chadwick's sign
   E. Quickening

4. A nurse in a prenatal clinic is caring for a client who is pregnant and experiencing episodes of hypotension. The client asks the nurse what causes these episodes. Which of the following responses should the nurse make?

   A. "This is due to an increase in blood volume."
   B. "This is due to pressure from the uterus on the diaphragm."
   C. "This is due to the weight of the uterus on the large blood vessels."
   D. "This is due to increased blood flow through the heart."

5. A nurse in a clinic receives a phone call from a client whose period is 1 week late and requests a pregnancy test. Which of the following information should the nurse provide to the client?

   A. "You should wait until 6 weeks after your last period to be tested."
   B. "You should not take any medications for 24 hours prior to the test."
   C. "You should not eat or drink for at least 8 hours before the test."
   D. "You should collect the urine from your first morning void."

PRACTICE Active Learning Scenario

A nurse is caring for a client who is in the fourth week of gestation. The client asks about skin and breast changes that can occur during pregnancy. What information should the nurse include when reinforcing teaching? Use the ATI Active Learning Template: Basic Concept to complete this item.

RELATED CONTENT: Describe at least three changes that occur to skin and breasts during pregnancy.

UNDERLYING PRINCIPLES: Describe the physiological basis for these changes.

Application Exercises Key

1. A. **CORRECT:** April 1 minus 3 months plus 7 days and 1 year equals an estimated date of delivery of January. 8.

   B. This is incorrect using Nägele's rule.

   C. This is incorrect using Nägele's rule.

   D. This is incorrect using Nägele's rule.

   Ⓝ *NCLEX® Connection: Health Promotion and Maintenance, Health Promotion/Disease Prevention*

2. A. **CORRECT:** T1 indicates the client has delivered one newborn at term.

   B. P0 indicates the client has had no preterm deliveries.

   C. A1 indicates the client has had one miscarriage.

   D. **CORRECT:** G3 indicates the client has had two prior pregnancies and the client is currently pregnant.

   E. **CORRECT:** L1 indicates the client has one living child.

   Ⓝ *NCLEX® Connection: Health Promotion and Maintenance, Data Collection Techniques*

3. A. Enlarged Montgomery glands are a presumptive sign of pregnancy.

   B. **CORRECT:** Goodell's sign is a probable sign of pregnancy.

   C. **CORRECT:** Ballottement is a probable sign of pregnancy.

   D. **CORRECT:** Chadwick's sign is a probable sign of pregnancy.

   E. Quickening is a presumptive sign of pregnancy.

   Ⓝ *NCLEX® Connection: Reduction of Risk Potential, Potential for Alterations in Body Systems*

4. A. An increase in blood volume during pregnancy results in cardiac hypertrophy.

   B. Pressure from the gravid uterus on the diaphragm can cause the client to experience shortness of breath.

   C. **CORRECT:** Maternal hypotension occurs when the client is lying in the supine position and the weight of the gravid uterus places pressure on the vena cava, decreasing venous blood flow to the heart.

   D. An increase in cardiac output during pregnancy results in cardiac hypertrophy.

   Ⓝ *NCLEX® Connection: Physiological Adaptation, Alterations in Body Systems*

5. A. The production of hCG can be detected about 8 days after conception.

   B. The nurse should not advise the client to stop taking medications in preparation for pregnancy tests. The nurse should review the client's medications to determine whether they can affect the results.

   C. The nurse should not advise the client to remain NPO prior to pregnancy testing. Serum or blood tests are not affected by food or fluid intake.

   D. **CORRECT:** Urine pregnancy tests should be done on a first-voided morning specimen to provide the most accurate results.

   Ⓝ *NCLEX® Connection: Health Promotion and Maintenance, Ante/Intra/Postpartum and Newborn Care*

PRACTICE Answer

Using the ATI Active Learning Template: Basic Concept

RELATED CONTENT
- Skin changes: hyperpigmentation; linea nigra; chloasma (mask of pregnancy) on the face; striae gravidarum (stretch marks), most pronounced on abdomen and thighs
- Breast changes: darkening of the areola, enlarged Montgomery glands, increase in size and heaviness, increased sensitivity

UNDERLYING PRINCIPLES: Increase in estrogen and progesterone occurring during pregnancy

Ⓝ *NCLEX® Connection: Health Promotion and Maintenance, Developmental Stages and Transitions*

UNIT 1   ANTEPARTUM NURSING CARE

SECTION: CHANGES DURING PREGNANCY

CHAPTER 3   *Prenatal Care*

Prenatal care involves data collection and reinforcement of education for expectant mothers. When providing prenatal care, nurses must take into account cultural considerations.

Prenatal education encompasses information provided to a client who is pregnant. Major areas of focus include assisting the client in self care of the discomforts of pregnancy, promoting a safe outcome to pregnancy, and fostering positive feelings by the client and family regarding the childbearing experience.

Prenatal care dramatically reduces infant and maternal morbidity and mortality rates by early detection and treatment of potential problems. A majority of birth defects occur between 2 and 8 weeks of gestation. Q͎ᴇʙᴘ

DATA COLLECTION

Nurses play an integral role in determining a client's current knowledge, previous pregnancies, and birthing experiences.

CLIENT HISTORY

- **Reproductive and obstetrical history** (contraception use, gynecological diagnoses, obstetrical difficulties)
- **Medical history**, including physical preexisting conditions, surgical procedures, any handicapping conditions, and immune status (rubella and hepatitis B)
- **Nutritional history**: A complete dietary assessment can alert the practitioner to deficient practices and food allergies. Good nutrition is important and has a direct effect on the growth and development of the fetus.
- **Family history** (genetic disorders, conditions that could affect the mother or fetus)
- Any recent or current illnesses or infections
- **Current medications**, including substance use and alcohol consumption. The nurse should display a nonjudgmental, matter-of-fact demeanor when interviewing a client regarding substance use and observe for findings such as lack of grooming.
- **Psychosocial history** (emotional response to pregnancy, adolescent pregnancy, partner, support system, history of depression, intimate partner violence issues)

- Any hazardous environmental exposures; current work conditions Qs
- Current exercise and lifestyle
- **Abuse history or risk**: Check all clients for all forms, including physical, sexual, or psychological abuse, because the risk increases during pregnancy.

BIRTH PLAN

Provide information about birthing methods, such as Lamaze, and pain control options (epidural, natural childbirth). Qᴘᴄᴄ

PRENATAL DATA COLLECTION

Prenatal care begins with an initial visit (within the first 12 weeks) and continues throughout pregnancy. In an uneventful pregnancy, prenatal visits are scheduled monthly for weeks 16 through 28, every 2 weeks from 29 through 36 weeks, and every week from 36 weeks until birth.

Initial prenatal visit

- Determine the estimated date of birth based on the last menstrual period.
- Obtain medical and nursing history to include social supports and review of systems (to determine risk factors).
- Collect baseline physical data including the client's baseline weight and vital signs
- Obtain initial laboratory tests, including hemoglobin, hematocrit, WCB, blood type and Rh, rubella titer, urinalysis, renal function test, Pap test, cervical cultures, HIV antibody, hepatitis B surface antigen, toxoplasmosis, and RPR or VDRL.

Ongoing prenatal visits

- Monitor weight, blood pressure, and urine for glucose, protein, and leukocytes.
- Monitor for edema.
- Monitor fetal development.
  - FHR can be detected at early appointments by ultrasound. The heartbeat can be heard by Doppler late in the first trimester. Listen at the midline, right above the symphysis pubis, by holding the Doppler firmly on the abdomen.
  - Measure fundal height starting in the second trimester. From weeks 18 to 30, the fundal height in centimeters is approximately the same as the number of weeks gestation.
  - Fetal health data collection: Begin checking for fetal movement between 16 and 20 weeks of gestation.
- Reinforce education for self-care to include management of common discomforts and concerns of pregnancy (nausea, vomiting, fatigue, backache, varicosities, heartburn, activity, sexuality).

Nursing care

- Assist with performing Leopold maneuvers to palpate presentation and position of the fetus.
- Assist the provider with the gynecological examination. This examination is performed to determine the status of a client's reproductive organs and birth canal. Pelvic measurements determine whether the pelvis will allow for the passage of the fetus at birth. Qᴛᴄ
  - The nurse has the client empty her bladder and take deep breaths during the examination to decrease discomfort.
- Administer Rho(D) immune globulin IM around 28 weeks of gestation for clients who are Rh-negative.

Routine laboratory tests

Blood type, Rh factor, and presence of irregular antibodies determine the risk for maternal-fetal blood incompatibility (erythroblastosis fetalis) or neonatal hyperbilirubinemia. Indirect Coombs test identifies clients sensitized to Rh-positive blood. For clients who are Rh-negative and not sensitized, the indirect Coombs test is repeated between 24 and 28 weeks of gestation.

CBC with differential, Hgb, and Hct detect infection and anemia.

Hgb electrophoresis identifies hemoglobinopathies (sickle cell anemia and thalassemia).

Rubella titer determines immunity to rubella.

Hepatitis B screen identifies carriers of hepatitis B.

Group B Streptococcus (GBS): Obtain a vaginal/anal culture at 35 to 37 weeks of gestation to check for GBS infection.

Urinalysis with microscopic examination of pH, specific gravity, color, sediment, protein, glucose, albumin, RBCs, WBCs, casts, acetone, and human chorionic gonadotropin identify pregnancy, diabetes mellitus, gestational hypertension, renal disease, and infection.

One-hour glucose tolerance (oral ingestion or IV administration of concentrated glucose with venous sample taken 1 hr later [fasting not necessary]) identifies hyperglycemia. Done at initial visit for at-risk clients and at 24 to 28 weeks of gestation for all pregnant women (greater than 140 mg/dL requires follow up).

Three-hour glucose tolerance (fasting overnight prior to oral ingestion or IV administration of concentrated glucose with a venous sample taken 1, 2, and 3 hr later) is used in clients who have elevated 1-hr glucose test as a screening tool for diabetes mellitus. A diagnosis of gestational diabetes requires two elevated blood-glucose readings.

Papanicolaou (Pap) test is used as a screening tool for cervical cancer, herpes simplex type 2, and human papillomavirus.

Vaginal/cervical culture detects streptococcus β-hemolytic, bacterial vaginosis, or sexually transmitted infections (gonorrhea, chlamydia).

PPD (tuberculosis screening), chest x-ray after 20 weeks of gestation with PPD test identifies exposure to tuberculosis.

Venereal disease research laboratory (VDRL): Syphilis screening mandated by law.

HIV: The enzyme immunoassay (EIA) test is a common test for initial HIV screening, with confirmation of a positive result by the Western blot or other secondary test. The Centers for Disease Control and Prevention and the American Congress of Obstetricians and Gynecologists recommend testing all clients who are pregnant unless the client refuses testing.

Toxoplasmosis, other infections, rubella, cytomegalovirus, and herpes virus (TORCH) screening when indicated: Screening for a group of infections capable of crossing the placenta and adversely affecting fetal development.

Maternal serum alpha-fetoprotein (MSAFP): Screening occurs at 15 to 22 weeks of gestation. Used to rule out Down syndrome (low level) and neural tube defects (high level). The provider might decide to use a more reliable indicator and opt for the Quad screen instead of the MSAFP at 16 to 18 weeks of gestation. This includes AFP, inhibin-A, a combination analysis of human chorionic gonadotropin, and estriol.

CLIENT EDUCATION

Prenatal education includes health promotion, preparation for pregnancy and birth, common discomforts of pregnancy, and findings of potential complications to report.

HEALTH PROMOTION

Preconception and prenatal education emphasizes healthy behaviors that promote the health of the pregnant client and fetus. Qᴘᴄᴄ

- Avoid all over-the-counter medications, supplements, and prescription medications unless the provider who is supervising care has knowledge of this practice.
- Alcohol (birth defects) and tobacco (low birth weight) are contraindicated during pregnancy.
- Substance use of any kind is to be avoided during pregnancy and lactation. The nurse should discuss strategies to reduce or eliminate substance use.
- Exercise during pregnancy yields positive benefits and should consist of 30 min of moderate exercise (walking or swimming) daily if not medically or obstetrically contraindicated.
- Avoid the use of hot tubs or saunas.
- Consume at least 8 glasses (2 L) of water each day.
- Get a flu immunization.
- Do not smoke.
- Treat current infections.
- Genetic testing and counseling are available.
- Avoid exposure to hazardous materials.

PREPARATION FOR PREGNANCY AND BIRTH

- Nurses provide anticipatory teaching to the client and family about the following.
  - Physical and emotional changes during pregnancy and interventions that can be implemented to provide relief
  - Indications of complications to report to the provider
  - Birthing options available to enhance the birthing process
- Maternal adaptation to pregnancy and the attainment of the maternal role—whereby the idea of pregnancy is accepted and assimilated into the client's way of life—includes hormonal and psychological aspects.
  - Emotional lability is experienced by many women with unpredictable mood changes and increased irritability, tearfulness, and anger alternating with feelings of joy and cheerfulness. This might result from hormonal changes.
  - A feeling of ambivalence about the pregnancy, which is a normal response, might occur early in the pregnancy and resolve before the third trimester. It consists of conflicting feelings (joy, pleasure, sorrow, hostility) about the pregnancy. These feelings can occur simultaneously, whether the pregnancy was planned or not.
- The nurse anticipates reviewing prenatal education topics with a client based on her current knowledge and previous pregnancy and birth experiences. The client's readiness to learn is enhanced when the nurse provides teaching during the appropriate trimester based on learning needs. Using a variety of educational methods (pamphlets, videos) and having the client verbalize and demonstrate learned topics ensure that learning has taken place. Qpcc

FIRST TRIMESTER

- Physical and psychosocial changes
- Common discomforts of pregnancy and measures to provide relief
- Lifestyle: exercise; stress; nutrition; dental care; over-the-counter and prescription medications; tobacco, alcohol, and substance use; sexual health and STIs (encourage safe sex practices)
- Possible complications and indications to report (preterm labor)
- Fetal growth and development
- Prenatal exercise
- Expected laboratory testing

SECOND TRIMESTER

- Benefits of breastfeeding
- Common discomforts and relief measures
- Lifestyle: sex and pregnancy, rest and relaxation, posture, body mechanics, clothing, seat belt safety and travel Qs
- Fetal movement
- Complications (preterm labor, gestational hypertension, gestational diabetes mellitus, premature rupture of membranes)

- Preparation for childbirth and childbirth education classes
- Review of birthing methods
- Development of a birth plan (verbal or written agreement about client wishes during labor and delivery)

THIRD TRIMESTER

- Childbirth preparation Qebp
  - Childbirth classes or birth plan
  - Coping methods
  - Breathing and relaxation techniques
  - Use of effleurage and counter pressure
  - Application of heat/cold, touch and massage, and water therapy
  - Use of transcutaneous electrical nerve stimulation (TENS)
  - Acupressure and acupuncture
  - Music and aromatherapy
  - Discussion regarding pain management during labor and birth (natural childbirth, epidural)
  - Use of doula during labor
  - Indications of term and preterm labor
  - Labor process
  - Infant care
  - Postpartum care
- Fetal movement/kick counts to ascertain fetal well-being: A client should be instructed to count and record fetal movements or kicks daily. There are several methods to complete kick counts.
  - In one method, clients count fetal activity two or three times a day for 2 hr after meals or bedtime. Fetal movements of less than three per hour or movements that cease entirely for 12 hr indicate a need for further evaluation.
- Diagnostic testing for fetal well-being (nonstress test, biophysical profile, ultrasound, contraction stress test)

COMMON DISCOMFORTS OF PREGNANCY

Nausea and vomiting commonly occur during the first trimester. The client should eat crackers or dry toast 30 min to 1 hr before rising in the morning to relieve discomfort. Instruct the client to avoid having an empty stomach and ingesting spicy, greasy, or gas-forming foods. Encourage the client to drink fluids between meals.

Breast tenderness can occur during the first trimester. The client should wear a bra that provides adequate support.

Urinary frequency can occur during the first and third trimesters. The client should empty her bladder frequently, decrease fluid intake before bedtime, and use perineal pads. The client is taught how to perform Kegel exercises (alternate tightening and relaxation of pubococcygeal muscles) to reduce stress incontinence (leakage of urine with coughing and sneezing).

Urinary tract infections (UTIs) are common during pregnancy because of renal changes and the vaginal flora becoming more alkaline.
- UTI risks can be decreased by encouraging the client to wipe the perineal area from front to back after voiding, avoiding bubble baths, wearing cotton underpants, avoiding tight-fitting pants, and consuming plenty of water (2 L per day). Q EBP
- The client should urinate before and after intercourse to flush bacteria from the urethra that are present or introduced during intercourse.
- Advise the client to urinate as soon as the urge occurs because retaining urine provides an environment for bacterial growth.
- Advise the client to notify the provider if urine is foul-smelling, contains blood, or appears cloudy.

Fatigue might occur during the first and third trimesters. The client is encouraged to engage in frequent rest periods.

Heartburn can occur during the second and third trimesters due to the stomach being displaced by the enlarging uterus and a slowing of gastrointestinal tract motility and digestion brought about by increased progesterone levels. The client should eat small, frequent meals; not allow the stomach to get too empty or too full; sit up for 30 min after meals; and check with the provider prior to using any over-the-counter antacids.

Constipation can occur during the second and third trimesters. The client is encouraged to drink plenty of fluids, eat a diet high in fiber, and exercise regularly.

Hemorrhoids can occur during the second and third trimesters. A warm sitz bath, witch hazel pads, and topical ointments will help relieve discomfort.

Backaches are common during the second and third trimesters. The client is encouraged to exercise regularly, perform pelvic tilt exercises (alternately arching and straightening the back), use proper body mechanics by using the legs to lift rather than the back, and use the side-lying position.

Shortness of breath and dyspnea can occur because of the enlarged uterus, which limits inspiration. The client should maintain good posture, sleep with extra pillows, and contact the provider if symptoms worsen.

Leg cramps during the third trimester can occur due to the compression of lower-extremity nerves and blood vessels by the enlarging uterus. This can result in poor peripheral circulation, as well as an imbalance in the calcium/phosphorus ratio. The client should extend the affected leg, keeping the knee straight, and dorsiflex the foot (toes toward head). Application of heat over the affected muscle or a foot massage while the leg is extended can help relieve cramping. The client should notify her provider if frequent cramping occurs.

Varicose veins and lower-extremity edema can occur during the second and third trimesters. The client should rest with legs elevated, avoid constricting clothing, wear support hose, avoid sitting or standing in one position for extended periods of time, and not sit with legs crossed at the knees. The client should sleep in the left-lateral position and exercise moderately with frequent walking to stimulate venous return.

Gingivitis, nasal stuffiness, and epistaxis (nosebleed) can occur as a result of elevated estrogen levels causing increased vascularity and proliferation of connective tissue. The client should gently brush teeth, observe good dental hygiene, use a humidifier, and use normal saline nose drops or spray.

Braxton Hicks contractions, which occur from the first trimester onward, can increase in intensity and frequency during the third trimester. A change of position and walking should cause contractions to subside. If contractions increase in intensity and frequency (true contractions) with regularity, the client should notify the provider.

Supine hypotension occurs when a client lies on her back and the weight of the gravid uterus compresses her vena cava. This reduces blood supply to the fetus. The client might experience feelings of lightheadedness and faintness. Teach the client to lie in a side-lying or semi-sitting position with knees slightly flexed.

DANGER SIGNS DURING PREGNANCY

The following indicate potential dangerous situations that should be reported to the provider immediately.

FIRST TRIMESTER
- Burning on urination (infection)
- Severe vomiting (hyperemesis gravidarum)
- Diarrhea (infection)
- Fever or chills (infection)
- Abdominal cramping and/or vaginal bleeding (miscarriage, ectopic pregnancy)

SECOND AND THIRD TRIMESTER
- Gush of fluid from the vagina (rupture of amniotic fluid) prior to 37 weeks of gestation
- Vaginal bleeding (placental problems such as abruption or previa)
- Abdominal pain (premature labor, abruptio placentae, ectopic pregnancy)
- Changes in fetal activity (decreased fetal movement can indicate fetal distress)
- Persistent vomiting (hyperemesis gravidarum)
- Severe headaches (gestational hypertension)
- Elevated temperature (infection)
- Dysuria (urinary tract infection)
- Blurred vision (gestational hypertension)
- Edema of face and hands (gestational hypertension)
- Epigastric pain (gestational hypertension)

Application Exercises

1. A nurse is reinforcing teaching with a group of clients about measures to relieve backache during pregnancy. Which of the following measures should the nurse include? (Select all that apply.)

   A. Avoid any lifting.

   B. Perform Kegel exercises twice a day.

   C. Perform the pelvic rock exercise every day.

   D. Use proper body mechanics.

   E. Avoid constrictive clothing.

2. A nurse is caring for a client who is pregnant and reviewing clinical manifestations of complications the client should promptly report to the provider. Which of the following complications should the nurse include?

   A. Vaginal bleeding

   B. Swelling of the ankles

   C. Heartburn after eating

   D. Lightheadedness when lying on her back

3. A client who is at 7 weeks of gestation is experiencing nausea and vomiting in the morning. Which of the following information should the nurse include?

   A. Eat crackers or plain toast before getting out of bed.

   B. Awaken during the night to eat a snack.

   C. Skip breakfast and eat lunch after nausea has subsided.

   D. Eat a large evening meal.

4. A nurse is discussing common discomforts of pregnancy with a client who is at 6 weeks of gestation. Which of the following findings should the nurse include? (Select all that apply.)

   A. Breast tenderness

   B. Urinary frequency

   C. Epistaxis

   D. Dysuria

   E. Epigastric pain

5. A client who is at 8 weeks of gestation tells the nurse that she isn't sure she is happy about being pregnant. Which of the following responses should the nurse make?

   A. "I will inform the provider that you are having these feelings."

   B. "It is normal to have these feelings during the first few months of pregnancy."

   C. "You should be happy that you are going to bring new life into the world."

   D. "I am going to make an appointment with the counselor for you to discuss these thoughts."

PRACTICE Active Learning Scenario

A nurse is caring for a client at 14 weeks of gestation and is reviewing self-care concepts regarding the prevention of urinary tract infections (UTIs). What should the nurse include in the teaching? Use the ATI Active Learning Template: Basic Concept to complete this item.

UNDERLYING PRINCIPLES: Describe two.

NURSING INTERVENTIONS: Describe two actions that decrease the risk of UTIs as they relate to each of the following types of interventions: When, why, and how?

Application Exercises Key

1. A. Lifting can be done by using the legs rather than the back.

   B. Kegel exercises are done to strengthen the perineal muscles and do not relieve backache.

   C. **CORRECT:** The pelvic rock or tilt exercise stretches the muscles of the lower back and helps relieve lower-back pain.

   D. **CORRECT:** The use of proper body mechanics prevents back injury due to the incorrect use of muscles when lifting.

   E. Avoiding constrictive clothing helps prevent urinary tract infections, vaginal infections, varicosities, and edema of the lower extremities.

   Ⓝ *NCLEX® Connection: Basic Care and Comfort, Nonpharmacological Comfort Interventions*

2. A. **CORRECT:** Vaginal bleeding indicates a potential complication of the placenta, such as placenta previa. The nurse should instruct the client to notify the provider immediately.

   B. Swelling of the ankles is common during pregnancy and can be relieved by sitting with the legs elevated.

   C. Heartburn occurs during pregnancy due to pressure on the stomach by the enlarging uterus. It can be relieved by eating small meals.

   D. Supine hypotension can be experienced by the client who feels lightheaded or faint when lying on her back. The nurse should instruct the client about the side-lying position to remove pressure of the uterus on the vena cava.

   Ⓝ *NCLEX® Connection: Physiological Adaptation, Alterations in Body Systems*

3. A. **CORRECT:** Nausea and vomiting during the first trimester can be relieved by eating crackers or plain toast 30 to 60 min prior to rising in the morning.

   B. Eating during the night can cause heartburn and does not relieve nausea and vomiting during the first trimester.

   C. Instruct the client to avoid an empty stomach for prolonged periods to reduce nausea and vomiting.

   D. Eating a large meal in the evening can cause heartburn and does not relieve morning nausea and vomiting.

   Ⓝ *NCLEX® Connection: Physiological Adaptation, Alterations in Body Systems*

4. A. **CORRECT:** Breast tenderness is a common discomfort occurring during the first trimester of pregnancy.

   B. **CORRECT:** Urinary frequency is a common discomfort occurring during the first trimester of pregnancy.

   C. **CORRECT:** Epistaxis is a common discomfort occurring during the first trimester of pregnancy.

   D. Dysuria is a complication that can occur during pregnancy. The nurse should instruct the client to report this finding to the provider.

   E. Epigastric pain is a clinical finding of preeclampsia. The nurse should instruct the client to report this finding to the provider.

   Ⓝ *NCLEX® Connection: Health Promotion and Maintenance, Developmental Stages and Transitions*

5. A. This is a nontherapeutic response by the nurse and does not acknowledge the client's concerns.

   B. **CORRECT:** Feelings of ambivalence about pregnancy are normal during the first trimester.

   C. This is a nontherapeutic response by the nurse and indicates disapproval.

   D. This is a nontherapeutic response by the nurse and does not acknowledge the client's feelings.

   Ⓝ *NCLEX® Connection: Health Promotion and Maintenance, Ante/Intra/Postpartum and Newborn Care*

PRACTICE Answer

Using ATI Active Learning Template: Basic Concept

UNDERLYING PRINCIPLES: UTIs are common because of renal changes during pregnancy and the vaginal flora becoming more alkaline.

NURSING INTERVENTIONS: Decrease risk of UTIs by:
- How, When: Encouraging client to wipe the perineal area from front to back after voiding.
- How: Avoiding bubble baths.
- How: Wearing cotton underpants; avoiding tight-fitting pants.
- How: Consuming at least 2 L of water per day.
- How, Why: Instructing client to urinate before and after intercourse to flush bacteria from the urethra that are present or introduced during intercourse.
- How, Why: Advising client to urinate as soon as the urge occurs because retaining urine provides an environment for bacterial growth.
- When, Why: Advising client to notify the provider if urine is foul-smelling, contains blood, or is cloudy so evaluation and early treatment can be initiated.

Ⓝ *NCLEX® Connection: Reduction of Risk Potential, Potential for Alterations in Body Systems*

CHAPTER 4

CHAPTER 4

Nutrition During Pregnancy

Adequate nutritional intake during pregnancy is essential to promoting fetal and maternal health.

Recommended weight gain during pregnancy, based on a single pregnancy, is usually 11.3 to 15.9 kg (25 to 35 lb). The general rule is that clients should gain 1 to 2 kg (2.2 to 4.4 lb) during the first trimester and approximately 0.4 kg (1 lb) per week for the last two trimesters. Underweight clients are advised to gain 28 to 40 lb; overweight clients, 15 to 25 lb.

It is important for the nurse to identify the client's nutritional choices, risk factors, and diet history. The nurse also should review specific nutritional guidelines for at-risk clients.

NURSING DATA COLLECTION AND INTERVENTIONS

DATA COLLECTION

Obtain subjective and objective dietary information.
- Journal of food habits, eating pattern, and cravings
- Nutrition-related questionnaires
- The client's weight on first prenatal visit and follow-up visits
- Laboratory findings (Hgb, iron levels)

Determine the client's caloric intake. Qpcc

Have the client record everything eaten during a 24-hr period. The nurse, dietitian, or client can identify the caloric value of each item. This record can provide better objective data about the client's nutrition status. **(4.1)**

CLIENT EDUCATION

Reinforce education about the following during pregnancy.
- **Increase calories:** An increase of 340 calories/day is recommended during the second trimester. An increase of 452 calories/day is recommended during the third trimester. If the client is breastfeeding during the postpartum period, additional caloric intake is advised. The American Academy of Pediatrics recommends that breastfeeding clients who are well nourished should add 450 to 500 calories/day to a balanced diet.
- **Increasing protein intake** is essential to basic growth.

- **Folic acid** is crucial for neurological development and the prevention of fetal neural tube defects. Foods high in folic acid include leafy vegetables, dried peas and beans, seeds, and orange juice. Breads, cereals, and other grains are fortified with folic acid. The March of Dimes recommends that clients who wish to become pregnant and clients of childbearing age take 400 mcg folic acid and clients who become pregnant take 600 mcg folic acid. Qebp
- **Iron supplements** are often added to the prenatal plan to facilitate an increase of the maternal RBC mass. Iron is best absorbed between meals and when given with a source of vitamin C. Milk and caffeine interfere with the absorption of iron supplements. Food sources of iron include beef liver, red meats, fish, poultry, dried peas and beans, and fortified cereals and breads. A stool softener might need to be added to decrease constipation experienced with iron supplements.
- **Calcium**, which is important to a developing fetus, is involved in bone and teeth formation. Sources of calcium include milk, calcium-fortified soy milk, fortified orange juice, nuts, legumes, and dark green leafy vegetables. Recommendation is 1,000 mg/day for pregnant and nonpregnant women 19 to 50 years of age, and 1,300 mg/day for those under 19 years of age.
- **Fluid:** 8 to 10 glasses (2.3 L) of fluid are recommended daily. Preferred fluids are water, fruit juice, and milk.
- **Limit caffeine:** The American Congress of Obstetricians and Gynecologists and March of Dimes recommend a daily intake of no more than 200 mg caffeine. The equivalent of 500 to 750 mL/day of coffee could increase the risk of a spontaneous abortion or fetal intrauterine growth restriction. Qebp
- It is recommended that women abstain from alcohol consumption during pregnancy.

4.1 Reviewing plan of care for a pregnant client

Expected outcomes

The client will consume the recommended dietary allowances/nutrients during her pregnancy.

Evaluation of the plan

Is there adequate weight gain?
Is the client compliant with the nursing plan of care?

Interventions

The nurse checks the client's dietary journal on the next prenatal visit.

The nurse provides educational materials regarding nutritional benefits to the mother and her newborn.

The nurse provides encouragement and answers questions that the client has regarding her dietary plans.

The nurse weighs the client and monitors for manifestations of inadequate weight gain.

The nurse should notify the charge nurse if a referral is needed.

RISK FACTORS

Age, culture, education, and socioeconomic issues could affect adequate nutrition during pregnancy. Some conditions specific to each client might inhibit adequate caloric intake.

- Adolescents can have poor nutritional habits (a diet low in vitamins and protein, not taking prescribed iron supplements).
- Vegetarians can have low protein, calcium, iron, zinc, and vitamin B_{12}.
- Nausea and vomiting during pregnancy
- Anemia
- Eating disorders (anorexia nervosa, bulimia nervosa)
- The appetite disorder pica (craving to eat nonfood substances such as dirt or red clay) can diminish the amount of nutritional foods ingested.
- Excessive weight gain can lead to macrosomia and labor complications.
- Inability to gain weight could result in low birth weight of the newborn.
- The nurse should advise clients who are financially unable to purchase/access food about the Women, Infants and Children (WIC) programs, which are federally funded state programs for pregnant women and children (up to 5 years old). Qᴛᴄ

DIETARY COMPLICATIONS DURING PREGNANCY

Nausea and constipation

Nausea and constipation are common during pregnancy.

- For nausea, tell the client to eat small amounts frequently (every 2 to 3 hr) to avoid large meals that distend the stomach and avoid alcohol, caffeine, and fried, fatty, and spicy foods. Also avoid consuming excessive amounts of fluid, and DO NOT take a medication to control nausea without first checking with the provider. Ginger (ginger ale soda, ginger tea, ginger candies) can also be helpful.
- For constipation, increase fluid consumption and include extra fiber in the diet. Fruits, vegetables, and whole grains contain fiber.

Diabetes mellitus

Preexisting diabetes mellitus and gestational diabetes mellitus are complications that require nutritional interventions.

- Monitor the amount of carbohydrates in the diet and keep glucose levels within target
- Limit the amount of sweets and desserts, which typically have large amounts of carbohydrates.
- Meet with a registered dietitian.

NUTRITION DURING POSTPARTUM

A lactating woman's nutritional plan includes the following instructions.

- Increase protein and calorie intake while adhering to a recommended, well-balanced diet.
- Increase oral fluids, but avoid alcohol and caffeine.
- Avoid food substances that do not agree with the newborn (foods that can cause altered bowel function).
- Take calcium supplements if consuming an inadequate amount of dietary calcium.

A nutritional plan for a woman who is not breastfeeding should include resumption of a previously recommended well-balanced diet.

Application Exercises

1. A nurse in a prenatal clinic is reinforcing education with a client who at 8 weeks of gestation. The client states that she does not like milk. Which of the following foods should the nurse recommend as a good source of calcium?

   A. Dark green leafy vegetables

   B. Deep red or orange vegetables

   C. White breads and rice

   D. Meat, poultry, and fish

2. A nurse in a prenatal clinic is caring for four clients. Which of the following clients' weight gain should the nurse report to the provider?

   A. 1.8 kg (4 lb) weight gain in the first trimester

   B. 3.6 kg (8 lb) weight gain in the first trimester

   C. 6.8 kg (15 lb) weight gain in the second trimester

   D. 11.3 kg (25 lb) weight gain in the third trimester

3. A nurse in a clinic is reinforcing instructions with a client of childbearing age about recommended folic acid supplements. Which of the following defects can occur in the neonate as a result of folic acid deficiency?

   A. Iron deficiency anemia

   B. Poor bone formation

   C. Macrosomic fetus

   D. Neural tube defects

4. A nurse is reviewing a prescription for iron supplements with a client who is at 8 weeks of gestation and has iron deficiency anemia. Which of the following beverages should the nurse instruct the client to take the iron supplements with?

   A. Ice water

   B. Low-fat or whole milk

   C. Tea or coffee

   D. Orange juice

5. A nurse is assisting the charge nurse with reviewing postpartum nutrition needs with a group of new mothers who are breastfeeding their newborns. Which of the following statements by a member of the group indicates an understanding of the teaching?

   A. "I wish I could have my morning coffee every day."

   B. "I should take folic acid to increase my milk supply."

   C. "I will continue adding 330 calories per day to my diet."

   D. "I will continue my calcium supplements because I don't like milk."

PRACTICE Active Learning Scenario

A nurse is assisting a charge nurse in a prenatal clinic with preparing an in-service education program for a group of newly licensed nurses about risk factors preventing adequate nutrition during pregnancy. What information should the nurse include in this presentation? Use the ATI Active Learning Template: Basic Concept to answer this item.

UNDERLYING PRINCIPLES
- Identify one that is age-related.
- Identify two that are related to culture/lifestyle.
- Identify one that is related to a socioeconomic factor.
- Identify two that are related to dietary complications during pregnancy.

NURSING INTERVENTIONS: Describe a federal program that is available to woman and children to provide nutrition support.

Application Exercises Key

1. A. **CORRECT:** Sources of calcium for bone and teeth formation include low-oxalate, dark green leafy vegetables (kale, artichokes, turnip greens).

   B. Deep red or orange vegetables are good sources of vitamins C and A.

   C. White breads and rice do not contain high levels of calcium.

   D. Meat, poultry, and fish are sources of protein but do not contain high levels of calcium.

   Ⓝ *NCLEX® Connection: Basic Care and Comfort, Nutrition and Oral Hydration*

2. A. This client has gained the appropriate weight of 3 to 4 lb for a client in the first trimester.

   B. **CORRECT:** This client has exceeded the expected 3- to 4-lb weight gain of the first trimester.

   C. This client has gained the appropriate weight of 3 to 4 lb in the first trimester and approximately 1 lb per week in the second trimester.

   D. This client is within the recommended weight gain of 25 to 35 lb by the third trimester.

   Ⓝ *NCLEX® Connection: Physiological Adaptation, Alterations in Body Systems*

3. A. Iron deficiency anemia is the result of a lack of iron-rich dietary sources, such as meat, chicken, and fish.

   B. Calcium deficiency can result in poor bone and teeth formation.

   C. Maternal obesity can lead to a macrosomic fetus.

   D. **CORRECT:** Neural tube defects are caused by folic acid deficiency. Food sources of folic acid include fresh green leafy vegetables, liver, peanuts, cereals, and whole-grain breads.

   Ⓝ *NCLEX® Connection: Basic Care and Comfort, Nutrition and Oral Hydration*

4. A. Water does not promote absorption of iron, but drinking plenty of water can prevent constipation, which is an adverse effect of iron supplements.

   B. Milk interferes with iron absorption.

   C. Caffeine, found in tea and coffee, can interfere with iron absorption. The client should consume no more than 200 mg/day because it increases the risk of spontaneous abortion or fetal intrauterine growth restriction.

   D. **CORRECT:** Orange juice contains vitamin C, which aids in the absorption of iron.

   Ⓝ *NCLEX® Connection: Pharmacological Therapies, Adverse Effects/ Contraindications/Side Effects/Interactions*

5. A. Women who are breastfeeding can have 1 to 2 cups of coffee or caffeinated beverage daily even though a minimal amount of caffeine enters breast milk and can affect the infant.

   B. Folic acid does not increase milk production.

   C. Women who are breastfeeding require an additional 450 to 500 calories per day to produce breast milk.

   D. **CORRECT:** Postpartum women who are at risk for inadequate dietary calcium should continue taking calcium supplements during lactation.

   Ⓝ *NCLEX® Connection: Health Promotion and Maintenance, Health Promotion/Disease Prevention*

PRACTICE Answer

Using the ATI Active Learning Template: Basic Concept

UNDERLYING PRINCIPLES
- Age-related: Adolescents can have poor nutritional habits during pregnancy.
- Culture/lifestyle
  - Vegetarians can have diets low in protein, calcium, zinc, and vitamin B_{12}.
  - Excessive weight gain can lead to macrosomia and labor complications.
- Socioeconomic: Inability to purchase or access foods can limit nutrition during pregnancy.
- Dietary complications: Nausea and vomiting during pregnancy, anemia, eating disorders (anorexia nervosa, bulimia nervosa), inability to gain weight, presence of the appetite disorder pica.

NURSING INTERVENTIONS: Women, Infants and Children (WIC) is a federally funded state program that provides nutritional support to pregnant women and their children (up to 5 years old).

Ⓝ *NCLEX® Connection: Health Promotion and Maintenance, Community Resources*

UNIT 1   ANTEPARTUM NURSING CARE
SECTION: CHANGES DURING PREGNANCY

CHAPTER 5 # Determination of Fetal Well-Being

Diagnostic procedures that determine fetal well-being include ultrasound (abdominal, transvaginal, Doppler), biophysical profile, nonstress test, contraction stress test, and amniocentesis. Additional diagnostic procedures include quad marker screening, and maternal serum alpha-fetoprotein (MSFAP).

Ultrasound (abdominal, transvaginal, Doppler)

Ultrasound is a procedure lasting approximately 20 min that consists of high-frequency sound waves used to visualize internal organs and tissues by producing a real-time, three-dimensional image of the developing fetus and maternal structures (fetal heart rate [FHR], pelvic anatomy). An ultrasound allows for early diagnosis of complications, permits earlier interventions, and thereby decreases neonatal and maternal morbidity and mortality. There are three types of ultrasound: external abdominal, transvaginal, and Doppler.

External abdominal ultrasound

A safe, noninvasive, painless procedure in which an ultrasound transducer is moved over the abdomen to obtain an image. An abdominal ultrasound is more useful after the first trimester when the gravid uterus is larger. The client should have a full bladder for the procedure during the first trimester. Qebp

Transvaginal ultrasound

An invasive procedure in which a probe is inserted vaginally to allow for a more accurate evaluation. An advantage of this procedure is that it does not require a full bladder.
- It is especially useful in clients who are obese and those in the first trimester to detect an ectopic pregnancy, identify abnormalities, and to establish gestational age.
- A transvaginal ultrasound also can be used in the third trimester in conjunction with abdominal scanning to evaluate for preterm labor.

Doppler ultrasound blood flow analysis

A noninvasive external ultrasound method to study the maternal-fetal blood flow by measuring the velocity at which RBCs travel in the uterine and fetal vessels using a handheld ultrasound device that reflects sound waves from a moving target. It is especially useful in fetal intrauterine growth restriction (IUGR) and poor placental perfusion, and as an adjunct in pregnancies at risk because of hypertension, diabetes mellitus, multiple fetuses, or preterm labor.

Two-dimensional (2D): standard medical scan; black, white, or shades of gray

Three-dimensional (3D): multiple pictures at once; almost as clear as a photograph; images look more lifelike than standard ultrasound images

Four-dimensional (4D): like 3D but also shows fetal movements in a video

INDICATIONS

POTENTIAL DIAGNOSES

- Confirming pregnancy
- Confirming gestational age by biparietal diameter (side-to-side) measurement
- Identifying multifetal pregnancy
- Determining site of fetal implantation (uterine, ectopic)
- Assessing fetal growth and development
- Assessing maternal structures
- Confirming fetal viability or death
- Ruling out or verifying fetal abnormalities
- Locating the site of placental attachment
- Determining amniotic fluid volume
- Observing fetal movement (fetal heartbeat, breathing, activity)
- Assessing fetal position
- Placental grading (evaluating placental maturation)
- Adjunct for other procedures (amniocentesis, biophysical profile)

CLIENT PRESENTATION

- Vaginal bleeding evaluation
- Questionable fundal height measurement in relationship to gestational weeks
- Reports of decreased fetal movements
- Preterm labor
- Questionable rupture of membranes

CONSIDERATIONS

NURSING ACTIONS

CLIENT PREPARATION

- Explain the procedure and that it presents no known risk to the client or the fetus.
- Advise the client to drink 1 quart of water prior to the ultrasound to fill the bladder if she is in the first trimester
- Assist the client into a supine position with a wedge placed under the right hip to displace the uterus (prevents supine hypotension). Qs

ONGOING CARE

- Allow the client to empty her bladder after the procedure.
- Provide the client with a washcloth or tissues to wipe away gel after completion of ultrasound.

Transvaginal ultrasound

CLIENT PREPARATION: Assist the client into a lithotomy position. The vaginal probe is covered with a protective device such as a condom, lubricated with a water-soluble gel, and inserted by the client or examiner.

ONGOING CARE

- During the procedure, the position of the probe or tilt of the table can be changed to facilitate the complete view of the pelvis.
- Inform the client that she might feel pressure as the probe is moved.

CLIENT EDUCATION

Fetal and maternal structures can be pointed out to the client as the ultrasound procedure is performed.

Biophysical profile

Biophysical profile (BPP) uses a real-time ultrasound to visualize physical and physiological characteristics of the fetus and observe for fetal biophysical responses to stimuli. It combines FHR monitoring (nonstress test) and fetal ultrasound.

INDICATIONS

POTENTIAL DIAGNOSES

- Nonreactive nonstress test
- Suspected oligohydramnios or polyhydramnios
- Suspected fetal hypoxemia or hypoxia

CLIENT PRESENTATION

- Premature rupture of membranes
- Maternal infection
- Decreased fetal movement
- IUGR

CONSIDERATIONS

NURSING ACTIONS: Prepare the client following the same nursing management principles as for an ultrasound.

INTERPRETATION OF FINDINGS

BPP assesses fetal well-being by measuring five variables with a score of 2 for each normal finding, and 0 for each abnormal finding for each variable.

VARIABLES

FHR
- Reactive (nonstress test) = 2
- Nonreactive = 0

Fetal breathing movements
- At least one episode of greater than 30 seconds duration in 30 min = 2
- Absent or less than 30 seconds duration = 0

Gross body movements
- At least three body or limb extensions with return to flexion in 30 min = 2
- Less than three episodes = 0

Fetal tone
- At least one episode of extension with return to flexion = 2
- Low extension and flexion, lack of flexion, or absent movement = 0

Qualitative amniotic fluid volume
- At least one pocket of fluid that measures at least 2 cm in two perpendicular planes = 2
- Pockets absent or less than 2 cm = 0

TOTAL SCORE FINDINGS

8 TO 10: **normal**, low risk of chronic fetal asphyxia

4 TO 6: **abnormal**, suspect chronic fetal asphyxia

LESS THAN 4: **abnormal**, strongly suspect chronic fetal asphyxia

Nonstress test

Nonstress test (NST) is the most widely used technique for antepartum evaluation of fetal well-being performed during the third trimester. It is a noninvasive procedure that monitors response of the FHR to fetal movement. A Doppler transducer (used to monitor FHR) and a tocotransducer (used to monitor uterine contractions) are attached externally to a client's abdomen to obtain tracing strips. The client can be asked to push a button whenever she feels a fetal movement, which is then noted on the tracing.

Disadvantages of an NST include a high rate of false nonreactive results with the fetal movement response blunted by sleep cycles of the fetus, fetal immaturity, maternal medications, and nicotine use disorder.

INDICATIONS

POTENTIAL DIAGNOSES

Checking for an intact fetal CNS during the third trimester

CLIENT PRESENTATION

- Decreased fetal movement
- Intrauterine growth restriction
- Postmaturity
- Gestational diabetes mellitus
- Gestational hypertension
- Maternal chronic hypertension
- History of previous fetal demise
- Advanced maternal age
- Sickle cell disease
- Isoimmunization

CONSIDERATIONS

NURSING ACTIONS

CLIENT PREPARATION

- Seat the client in a reclining chair, or place in a semi-Fowler's or left-lateral position.
- Apply conduction gel to the abdomen.
- Apply two belts to the abdomen, and attach the FHR and uterine contraction monitors.

ONGOING CARE

- Instruct the client to press the button on the handheld event marker each time she feels the fetus move.
- If there are no fetal movements (fetus sleeping), vibroacoustic stimulation (sound source, usually laryngeal stimulator) can be activated for 3 seconds on the maternal abdomen over the fetal head to awaken the sleeping fetus.

INTERPRETATION OF FINDINGS

- The NST is interpreted as reactive if the FHR is a normal baseline rate with moderate variability, accelerates at least 15/min above baseline (10/min above baseline prior to 32 weeks) for at least 15 seconds (10 seconds prior to 32 weeks) and occurs two or more times during a 20-min period. **(5.1)**
- Nonreactive NST is a test that does not demonstrate at least two qualifying accelerations in a 20-min window. If this is so, a further assessment (contraction stress test [CST], BPP) is indicated.

Contraction stress test

Nipple-stimulated contraction test

Consists of a client lightly brushing her palm across her nipple for 2 min, which causes the pituitary gland to release endogenous oxytocin, and then stopping the nipple stimulation when a contraction begins. The same process is repeated after a 5-min rest period.

- Analysis of the FHR response to contractions (which decrease placental blood flow) determines how the fetus will tolerate the stress of labor. A pattern of at least three contractions within a 10-min time period with duration of 40 to 60 seconds each must be obtained to use for assessment data.
- Hyperstimulation of the uterus (uterine contraction longer than 90 seconds or five or more contractions in 10 min) should be avoided by stimulating the nipple intermittently with rest periods in between and avoiding bimanual stimulation of both nipples unless stimulation of one nipple is unsuccessful.

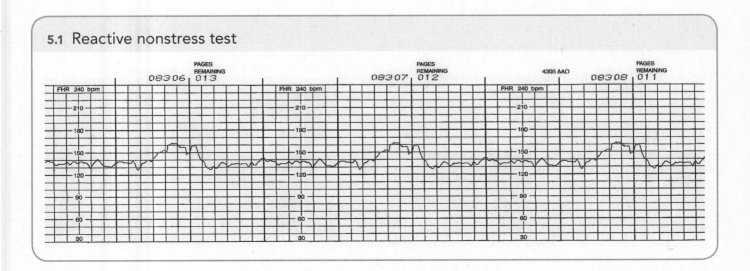

5.1 Reactive nonstress test

INDICATIONS

POTENTIAL DIAGNOSES

- High-risk pregnancies (gestational diabetes mellitus, postterm pregnancy)
- Nonreactive stress test

CLIENT PRESENTATION

- Decreased fetal movement
- Intrauterine growth restriction
- Postmaturity
- Gestational diabetes mellitus
- Gestational hypertension
- Maternal chronic hypertension
- History of previous fetal demise
- Advanced maternal age
- Sickle-cell disease

CONSIDERATIONS

NURSING ACTIONS

CLIENT PREPARATION
- Obtain and document a baseline of the FHR, fetal movement, and contractions for 10 to 20 min.
- Assist with obtaining informed consent. Qpcc

ONGOING CARE
- Initiate nipple stimulation if there are no contractions. Instruct the client to roll a nipple between her thumb and fingers or brush her palm across her nipple. The client should stop when a uterine contraction begins.
- Monitor and provide adequate rest periods for the client to avoid hyperstimulation of the uterus.

INTERVENTIONS
If hyperstimulation of the uterus or preterm labor occurs, do the following. QEBP
- Monitor for contractions lasting longer than 90 seconds or occurring more frequently than every 2 min.
- Administer tocolytics.
- Maintain bed rest during the procedure.
- Observe for 30 min afterward to see that contractions have ceased and preterm labor does not begin.

INTERPRETATION OF FINDINGS

NEGATIVE CST (NORMAL FINDING): Indicated if within a 10-min period, with three uterine contractions, there are no late decelerations of the FHR.

POSITIVE CST (ABNORMAL FINDING): Indicated with persistent and consistent late decelerations with 50% or more of the contractions. This is suggestive of uteroplacental insufficiency. Variable deceleration can indicate cord compression, and early decelerations can indicate fetal head compression. Based on these findings, the provider may determine to induce labor or perform a cesarean birth. **(5.2)**

COMPLICATIONS

Potential for preterm labor

Amniocentesis

The aspiration of amniotic fluid for analysis by insertion of a needle transabdominally into a client's uterus and amniotic sac under direct ultrasound guidance locating the placenta and determining the position of the fetus. It may be performed after 14 weeks of gestation.

INDICATIONS

POTENTIAL DIAGNOSES

- Previous birth with a chromosomal anomaly
- A parent who is a carrier of a chromosomal anomaly
- Family history of neural tube defects
- Prenatal diagnosis of a genetic disorder or congenital anomaly of the fetus
- Alpha-fetoprotein (AFP) level for fetal abnormalities
- Lung maturity assessment
- Fetal hemolytic disease
- Meconium in the amniotic fluid

CONSIDERATIONS

PREPROCEDURE

NURSING ACTIONS: Assist in obtaining informed consent.

CLIENT EDUCATION: Empty the bladder prior to the procedure to reduce its size and reduce the risk of inadvertent puncture. Qs

INTRAPROCEDURE

NURSING ACTIONS
- Obtain and document baseline vital signs and FHR prior to the procedure.
- Assist the client into a supine position. Place a wedge under the right hip to displace the uterus off the vena cava. Place a drape over the client, exposing only her abdomen.
- Prepare the client for an ultrasound to locate the placenta.
- Cleanse the abdomen with an antiseptic solution prior to the administration of a local anesthetic by the provider.

CLIENT EDUCATION: The client will feel slight pressure as the needle is inserted. Continue breathing, because holding the breath will lower the diaphragm against the uterus and shift the intrauterine contents.

5.2 Positive CST

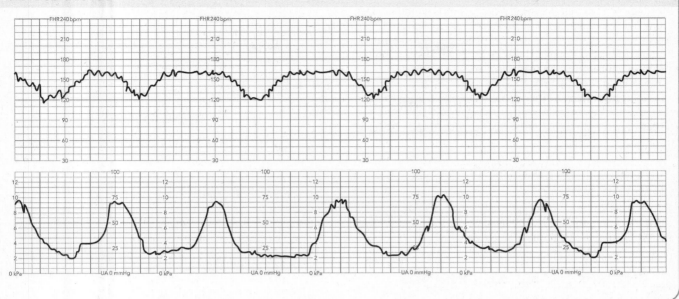

POSTPROCEDURE

NURSING ACTIONS
- Monitor vital signs, FHR, and uterine contractions throughout and 30 min following the procedure.
- Have the client rest for 30 min.
- Administer Rho(D) immune globulin to the client if she is Rh-negative (standard practice after an amniocentesis for all clients who are Rh-negative to protect against Rh isoimmunization). Q EBP

CLIENT EDUCATION
- Report to the provider of fever, chills, leakage of fluid or bleeding from the insertion site, decreased fetal movement, vaginal bleeding, or uterine contractions after the procedure.
- Drink plenty of liquids and rest for 24 hr postprocedure.

INTERPRETATION OF FINDINGS

AFP can be measured from the amniotic fluid between 15 and 20 weeks (16 to 18 weeks of gestation is ideal) and can be used to check for neural tube defects in the fetus or chromosomal disorders. Can be evaluated to follow up a high level of AFP in maternal serum.

HIGH LEVELS: Associated with neural tube defects (anencephaly [incomplete development of fetal skull and brain], spina bifida [open spine], omphalocele [abdominal wall defect]). High AFP levels also can be present with normal multifetal pregnancies.

LOW LEVELS: Associated with chromosomal disorders (Down syndrome) or gestational trophoblastic disease (hydatidiform mole).

Fetal lung tests

Tests for fetal lung maturity can be performed if gestation is less than 37 weeks, in the event of a rupture of membranes, for preterm labor, or for a complication indicating a cesarean birth. Amniotic fluid is tested to determine whether the fetal lungs are mature enough to adapt to extrauterine life, or if the fetus will likely have respiratory distress. Determination is made whether the fetus should be delivered immediately or if the fetus requires more time in utero with the administration of glucocorticoids to promote fetal lung maturity.

LECITHIN/SPHINGOMYELIN (L/S) RATIO: A 2:1 ratio indicates fetal lung maturity (2.5:1 or 3:1 for a client who has diabetes mellitus).

PHOSPHATIDYLGLYCEROL: Absence of phosphatidylglycerol is associated with respiratory distress.

COMPLICATIONS

- Amniotic fluid emboli
- Maternal or fetal hemorrhage
- Fetomaternal hemorrhage with Rh isoimmunization
- Maternal or fetal infection
- Inadvertent fetal damage or anomalies involving limbs
- Fetal death
- Inadvertent maternal intestinal or bladder damage
- Miscarriage or preterm labor
- Premature rupture of membranes
- Leakage of amniotic fluid

NURSING ACTIONS

- Monitor vital signs, temperature, respiratory status, FHR, uterine contractions, and vaginal discharge for amniotic fluid or bleeding.
- Administer medication.
- Offer support and reassurance.

Quad marker screening

This blood test ascertains information about the likelihood of fetal birth defects but does not diagnose the actual defect. It can be performed instead of the maternal serum AFP yielding more reliable findings. Includes testing for:
- **Human chorionic gonadotropin (hCG):** a hormone produced by the placenta
- **Alpha-fetoprotein (AFP):** a protein produced by the fetus
- **Estriol:** a protein produced by the fetus and placenta
- **Inhibin A:** a protein produced by the ovaries and placenta

INDICATIONS

CLIENT PRESENTATION
- Preferred at 16 to 18 weeks gestation
- Risk for giving birth to a neonate who has a genetic chromosomal abnormality

INTERPRETATION OF FINDINGS

- Low levels of AFP can indicate a risk for Down syndrome.
- High levels of AFP can indicate a risk for neural tube defects.
- Levels higher than the expected reference range of hCG and inhibin A indicates a risk for Down syndrome.
- Levels lower than the expected reference range of estriol can indicate a risk for Down syndrome.

Maternal serum alpha-fetoprotein

A screening tool used to detect neural tube defects. Clients who have abnormal findings should be referred for a quad marker screening, genetic counseling, ultrasound, and an amniocentesis.

INDICATIONS

All pregnant clients, preferably between 16 and 18 weeks of gestation

CONSIDERATIONS

PREPROCEDURE NURSING ACTIONS
- Discuss testing with the client.
- Draw blood sample.
- Offer support and education as needed.

INTERPRETATION OF FINDINGS

- High levels can indicate a neural tube defect or open abdominal defect.
- Low levels can indicate Down syndrome.

Application Exercises

1. A nurse is reviewing findings of a client's biophysical profile (BPP) with the charge nurse. Which of the following variables should the nurse expect the test to include? (Select all that apply.)

   A. Fetal weight

   B. Fetal breathing movement

   C. Fetal tone

   D. Fetal position

   E. Amniotic fluid volume

2. A nurse is assisting with the care of a client who is in preterm labor and is scheduled to undergo an amniocentesis. The nurse should review which of the following tests to determine fetal lung maturity?

   A. Alpha-fetoprotein (AFP)

   B. Lecithin/sphingomyelin (L/S) ratio

   C. Kleihauer-Betke test

   D. Indirect Coombs test

3. A nurse is assisting with the care of a client who is pregnant and undergoing a nonstress test. The nurse asks why the charge nurse is using a vibroacoustic stimulation device. Which of the following responses should the charge nurse make?

   A. "It is used to stimulate uterine contractions."

   B. "It will decrease the incidence of uterine contractions."

   C. "It lulls the fetus to sleep."

   D. "It awakens a sleeping fetus."

4. A nurse is reinforcing teaching with a client who is pregnant about the amniocentesis procedure. Which of the following statements should the nurse make?

   A. "You will lay on your right side during the procedure."

   B. "You should not eat anything for 24 hours prior to the procedure."

   C. "You should empty your bladder prior to the procedure."

   D. "The test is done to determine gestational age."

5. A nurse is assisting with the care of a client who is pregnant and is to undergo a contraction stress test (CST). Which of the following findings are indications for this procedure? (Select all that apply.)

   A. Decreased fetal movement

   B. Intrauterine growth restriction (IUGR)

   C. Postmaturity

   D. Placenta previa

   E. Amniotic fluid emboli

PRACTICE Active Learning Scenario

A nurse in a prenatal clinic is assisting with the orientation of a newly licensed nurse and discussing how to perform a nonstress test (NST). What should the nurse include in the discussion about the procedure? Use the ATI Active Learning Template: Diagnostic Procedure to complete this item.

INDICATIONS: Identify three that relate to the status of the fetus.

INTERPRETATION OF FINDINGS: Describe a nonreactive NST.

NURSING INTERVENTIONS: Include two preprocedure and one intraprocedure.

Application Exercises Key

1. A. Fetal weight is not one of the variables included in the BPP.
   B. **CORRECT:** Fetal breathing movements are included in the BPP.
   C. **CORRECT:** Fetal tone is included in the BPP.
   D. Fetal position is not included in the BPP.
   E. **CORRECT:** Amniotic fluid volume is included in the BPP.

   Ⓝ *NCLEX® Connection: Reduction of Risk Potential, Diagnostic Tests*

2. A. AFP is a test to assess for fetal neural tube defects or chromosome disorders.
   B. **CORRECT:** A test of the L/S ratio is done as a part of an amniocentesis to determine fetal lung maturity.
   C. A Kleihauer-Betke test is used to verify that fetal blood is present during a percutaneous umbilical blood sampling procedure.
   D. An indirect Coombs' test detects Rh antibodies in the mother's blood.

   Ⓝ *NCLEX® Connection: Reduction of Risk Potential, Diagnostic Tests*

3. A. The acoustic vibration device does not stimulate the uterus.
   B. The acoustic vibration device has no effect on the uterine muscles.
   C. The acoustic vibration device stimulates a sleeping fetus.
   D. **CORRECT:** The acoustic vibration device is activated for 3 seconds on the maternal abdomen over the fetal head to awaken a sleeping fetus.

   Ⓝ *NCLEX® Connection: Reduction of Risk Potential, Diagnostic Tests*

4. A. Assist the client into a supine position, place a wedge under her right hip to displace the uterus off the vena cava, and place a drape over the client, exposing only her abdomen.
   B. The client does not need to be NPO for 24 hr prior to the procedure.
   C. **CORRECT:** The client's bladder should be empty to avoid an inadvertent puncture during the procedure.
   D. Amniotic fluid is tested to identify fetal genetic defects. An amniocentesis does not determine gestational age.

   Ⓝ *NCLEX® Connection: Reduction of Risk Potential, Diagnostic Tests*

5. A. **CORRECT:** Decreased fetal movement is an indication for a CST.
   B. **CORRECT:** IUGR is an indication for a CST.
   C. **CORRECT:** Postmaturity is an indication for a CST.
   D. Placenta previa is a contraindication of a CST.
   E. Amniotic fluid emboli are a complication of an amniocentesis.

   Ⓝ *NCLEX® Connection: Reduction of Risk Potential, Diagnostic Tests*

PRACTICE Answer

Using the ATI Active Learning Template: Diagnostic Procedure

INDICATIONS
- Assessment for intact fetal CNS during the third trimester
- Decreased fetal movement
- Intrauterine growth restriction
- Postmaturity

INTERPRETATION OF FINDINGS:
Nonreactive NST is a test that does not demonstrate at least two qualifying accelerations in a 20-min window. If this is so, a further assessment, such as a contraction stress test or biophysical profile, is indicated.

NURSING INTERVENTIONS
- Preprocedure
  - Seat the client in a reclining chair in a semi-Fowler's or left-lateral position.
  - Apply conduction gel to the client's abdomen.
  - Apply the Doppler transducer and the tocotransducer.
- Intraprocedure: Instruct the client to depress the event marker button each time she feels fetal movement.

Ⓝ *NCLEX® Connection: Reduction of Risk Potential, Diagnostic Tests*

CHAPTER 6 **Bleeding During Pregnancy**

Vaginal bleeding during pregnancy is always abnormal and must be investigated to determine the cause. It can impair the outcome of the pregnancy and the mother's life. (6.1)

Spontaneous abortion

Spontaneous abortion is when a pregnancy is terminated before 20 weeks of gestation (the point of fetal viability) or a fetal weight less than 500 g.

Types of abortion are classified according to manifestations and whether the products of conception are partially or completely retained or expulsed. Types of abortions include **threatened**, **inevitable**, **incomplete**, **complete**, and **missed**.

DATA COLLECTION

RISK FACTORS

- Chromosomal abnormalities (account for 50%)
- Maternal illness, such as type 1 diabetes mellitus
- Advanced maternal age
- Premature cervical dilation
- Chronic maternal infections
- Maternal malnutrition
- Trauma or injury
- Anomalies in the fetus or placenta
- Substance use
- Antiphospholipid syndrome

EXPECTED FINDINGS (6.2)

- Backache and abdominal tenderness
- Rupture of membranes
- Dilation of the cervix
- Fever
- Manifestations of hemorrhage (hypotension, tachycardia)

LABORATORY TESTS

Hgb and Hct, if considerable blood loss

Clotting factors monitored for disseminated intravascular coagulopathy (DIC): a complication with retained products of conception

WBC for suspected infection

Serum human chorionic gonadotropin (hCG) levels to confirm pregnancy

DIAGNOSTIC AND THERAPEUTIC PROCEDURES

Ultrasound to determine the presence of a viable or dead fetus, or partial or complete products of conception within the uterine cavity

Examination of the cervix to observe whether it is opened or closed

Dilation and curettage (D&C) to dilate and scrape the uterine walls to remove uterine contents for inevitable and incomplete abortions

Dilation and evacuation (D&E) to dilate and evacuate uterine contents after 16 weeks of gestation

Prostaglandins and oxytocin to augment or induce uterine contractions and expel the products of conception

---

6.1 Causes of bleeding during pregnancy

First trimester

SPONTANEOUS ABORTION: Vaginal bleeding, uterine cramping, and partial or complete expulsion of products of conception

ECTOPIC PREGNANCY: Abrupt unilateral lower-quadrant abdominal pain with or without vaginal bleeding

Second trimester

GESTATIONAL TROPHOBLASTIC DISEASE: Uterine size increasing abnormally fast, abnormally high levels of hCG, nausea and increased emesis, no fetus present on ultrasound, and scant or profuse dark brown or red vaginal bleeding

Third trimester

PLACENTA PREVIA: Painless vaginal bleeding

ABRUPTIO PLACENTAE: Vaginal bleeding, sharp abdominal pain, and tender rigid uterus

VASA PREVIA: Fetal vessels are implanted into the membranes rather than the placenta.

Other causes of bleeding

RECURRENT PREMATURE DILATION OF THE CERVIX: Painless bleeding with cervical dilation leading to fetal expulsion

PRETERM LABOR: Pink-stained vaginal discharge, uterine contractions becoming regular, cervical dilation and effacement

---

PATIENT-CENTERED CARE

NURSING CARE

- Perform a pregnancy test.
- Observe color and amount of bleeding (count pads).
- Maintain client on bed rest. Inform client of risk for falls due to sedative medications if prescribed. Qs
- Avoid vaginal exams.
- Assist with an ultrasound.
- Administer medications and monitor blood products transfusions.
- Determine how much tissue has passed and save passed tissue for examination.
- Assist with termination of pregnancy (D&C, D&E, prostaglandin administration) as indicated.
- Use the lay term "miscarriage" with clients because the medical term "abortion" can be misunderstood.
- Provide information to client and partner about pregnancy loss support groups.
- Provide referral for client and partner to pregnancy loss support groups.

MEDICATIONS

- Analgesics and sedatives
- Prostaglandin as a vaginal suppository
- Oxytocin
- Broad-spectrum antibiotics, in septic abortion
- Rho(D) immune globulin in clients who are Rh-negative

CLIENT EDUCATION

- Notify the provider of heavy, bright red vaginal bleeding; elevated temperature; or foul-smelling vaginal discharge.
- A small amount of discharge is expected for 1 to 2 weeks.
- Take prescribed antibiotics.
- Refrain from tub baths, sexual intercourse, and placing anything into the vagina for 2 weeks.
- Avoid becoming pregnant for 2 months.

Ectopic pregnancy

Ectopic pregnancy is the abnormal implantation of a fertilized ovum outside of the uterine cavity, usually in the fallopian tube, which can result in a tubal rupture causing a fatal hemorrhage.

Ectopic pregnancy is the second most frequent cause of bleeding in early pregnancy and a leading cause of infertility.

DATA COLLECTION

RISK FACTORS

Any factor that compromises tubal patency (STIs, assisted reproductive technologies, tubal surgery, and contraceptive intrauterine device [IUD])

EXPECTED FINDINGS

- Unilateral stabbing pain and tenderness in the lower-abdominal quadrant
- Delayed (1 to 2 weeks), lighter than usual, or irregular menses
- Scant, dark red, or brown vaginal spotting that occurs 6 to 8 weeks after last normal menses; red, vaginal bleeding if rupture has occurred
- Referred shoulder pain due to blood in the peritoneal cavity irritating the diaphragm or phrenic nerve after tubal rupture
- Report of indications of shock (faintness, dizziness) related to amount of bleeding in abdominal cavity
- Manifestations of hemorrhage and shock (hypotension, tachycardia, pallor)

LABORATORY TESTS

Elevated hCG levels and a low progesterone level are indications of an ectopic pregnancy.

6.2 Types of spontaneous abortion

	CRAMPS	BLEEDING	TISSUE PASSED	CERVICAL OPENING
THREATENED	Possible mild cramps	Spotting to moderate	None	Closed
INEVITABLE	Moderate	Mild to severe	None	Dilated with membranes or tissue bulging at cervix
INCOMPLETE	Severe	Heavy, profuse	Partial fetal tissue or placenta	Dilated with tissue in cervical canal or passage of tissue
COMPLETE	Mild	Minimal	Complete expulsion of uterine contents	Closed with no tissue in cervical canal
MISSED	None	None; brownish discharge	None, prolonged retention of tissue	Closed
SEPTIC	Varies	Varies; malodorous discharge	Varies	Usually dilated
RECURRENT	Varies	Varies	Yes	Usually dilated

DIAGNOSTIC AND THERAPEUTIC PROCEDURES

Transvaginal ultrasound shows an empty uterus.

RAPID TREATMENT
- **Medical management** if rupture has not occurred and tube preservation desired.
- **Methotrexate** inhibits cell division and embryo enlargement, dissolving the pregnancy
- **Salpingostomy** is done to salvage the fallopian tube if not ruptured.
- **Laparoscopic salpingectomy** (removal of the tube) is performed when the tube has ruptured.

PATIENT-CENTERED CARE

NURSING CARE

- Replace fluids, and maintain electrolyte balance.
- Reinforce client education and provide psychological support.
- Administer medications.
- Prepare the client for surgery and postoperative nursing care.
- Provide information to the client and partner about pregnancy loss support groups.
- Obtain serum hCG and progesterone levels, liver and renal function studies, CBC, and type and Rh.

CLIENT EDUCATION

- If taking methotrexate, avoid alcohol consumption and vitamins containing folic acid to prevent a toxic response to the medication. Qs
- Protect against sun exposure (photosensitivity).

Gestational trophoblastic disease

Gestational trophoblastic disease (GTD) is the proliferation and degeneration of trophoblastic villi in the placenta that becomes swollen, fluid-filled, and takes on the appearance of grape-like clusters. The embryo fails to develop beyond a primitive state and these structures are associated with choriocarcinoma, which is a rapidly metastasizing malignancy. Two types of molar growths are identified by chromosomal analysis.

Complete mole

- All genetic material is paternally derived.
- The ovum has no genetic material, or the material is inactive.
- The complete mole contains no fetus, placenta, amniotic membranes, or fluid.
- There is no placenta to receive maternal blood. Hemorrhage into the uterine cavity occurs, and vaginal bleeding results.
- Approximately 20% of complete moles progress toward a choriocarcinoma.

Partial mole

- Genetic material is derived both maternally and paternally.
- A normal ovum is fertilized by two sperm or one sperm in which meiosis or chromosome reduction and division did not occur.
- A partial mole often contains abnormal embryonic or fetal parts, an amniotic sac, and fetal blood, but congenital anomalies are present.
- Approximately 6% of partial moles progress toward a choriocarcinoma.

DATA COLLECTION

RISK FACTORS

- Prior molar pregnancy
- Age early teens or older than age 40

EXPECTED FINDINGS

Excessive vomiting (hyperemesis gravidarum) due to elevated hCG levels

PHYSICAL FINDINGS
- Rapid uterine growth more than expected for the duration of the pregnancy due to the overproliferation of trophoblastic cells
- Bleeding is often dark brown resembling prune juice, or bright red that is either scant or profuse and continues for a few days or intermittently for a few weeks and can be accompanied by passage of vesicles.
- Anemia from blood loss
- Manifestations of preeclampsia that occur prior to 24 weeks of gestation

LABORATORY TESTS

Serum level of hCG persistently high compared with expected decline after weeks 10 to 12 of pregnancy

DIAGNOSTIC AND THERAPEUTIC PROCEDURES

- An ultrasound reveals a dense growth with characteristic vesicles, but no fetus in utero.
- Suction curettage is done to aspirate and evacuate the mole.
- Following mole evacuation, the client should undergo a baseline pelvic exam and ultrasound scan of the abdomen.
- Serum hCG analysis following molar pregnancy to be done weekly for 3 weeks, then monthly for 6 months to 1 year to detect GTD.

PATIENT-CENTERED CARE

NURSING CARE

- Measure fundal height.
- Monitor vaginal bleeding and discharge.
- Monitor gastrointestinal status and appetite.
- Monitor for manifestations of preeclampsia.
- Administer medications.
  - Rho(D) immune globulin to the client who is Rh-negative
  - Chemotherapeutic medications for manifestations of malignant cells indicating choriocarcinoma

CLIENT EDUCATION

- Save clots or tissue for evaluation.
- Provide emotional support.
- Information about pregnancy loss support groups.
- Use reliable contraception as a component of follow-up care.
- Follow-up is important due to the increased risk of choriocarcinoma.

Placenta previa

Placenta previa occurs when the placenta abnormally implants in the lower segment of the uterus near or over the cervical os instead of attaching to the fundus. The abnormal implantation results in bleeding during the third trimester of pregnancy as the cervix begins to dilate and efface. **(6.3)**

Classified into three types depending on the degree to which the cervical os is covered by the placenta

- **Complete or total:** The cervical os is completely covered by the placental attachment.
- **Incomplete or partial:** The cervical os is only partially covered by the placental attachment.
- **Marginal or low-lying:** The placenta is attached in the lower uterine segment but does not reach the cervical os.

DATA COLLECTION

RISK FACTORS

- Previous placenta previa
- Uterine scarring (previous cesarean birth, curettage, endometritis)
- Maternal age greater than 35 years
- Multifetal gestation
- Multiple gestations or closely spaced pregnancies
- Cigarette smoking

EXPECTED FINDINGS

- Painless, bright red vaginal bleeding during the second or third trimester
- Uterus soft, relaxed, and nontender with normal tone
- Fundal height greater than usually expected for gestational age
- Fetus in a breech, oblique, or transverse position
- Reassuring FHR
- Vital signs within normal limits
- Decreasing urinary output can be a better indicator of blood loss

LABORATORY TESTS

- CBC
- Blood type and Rh
- Coagulation profile
- Kleihauer-Betke test (used to detect fetal blood in maternal circulation)

DIAGNOSTIC PROCEDURES

- Transabdominal or transvaginal ultrasound for placement of the placenta
- Fetal monitoring for determination of fetal well-being

PATIENT-CENTERED CARE

NURSING CARE

- Monitor for bleeding, leakage, or contractions.
- Measure fundal height.
- Refrain from performing vaginal exams (can exacerbate bleeding). Qs
- Administer medications. Monitor IV fluids and blood products. Corticosteroids, such as betamethasone, promote fetal lung maturation if early delivery is anticipated (cesarean birth).
- Have oxygen equipment available in case of fetal distress.

CLIENT EDUCATION

- Maintain bed rest.
- Do not insert anything vaginally.

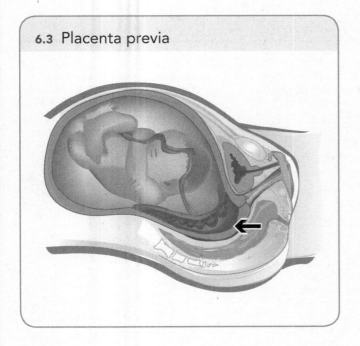

6.3 Placenta previa

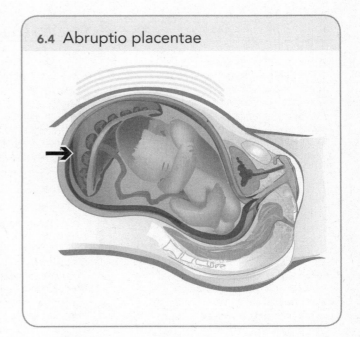

6.4 Abruptio placentae

Abruptio placentae

Abruptio placentae is the premature separation of the placenta from the uterus, which can be a partial or complete detachment. This separation occurs after 20 weeks of gestation, usually in the third trimester. It has significant maternal and fetal morbidity and mortality and is a leading cause of maternal death. **(6.4)**

Coagulation defect, such as disseminated intravascular coagulopathy (DIC), is often associated with moderate to severe abruption.

DATA COLLECTION

RISK FACTORS

- Maternal hypertension (chronic or gestational)
- Blunt external abdominal trauma (motor-vehicle crash, maternal battering)
- Cocaine use resulting in vasoconstriction
- Previous incidents of abruptio placentae
- Cigarette smoking
- Premature rupture of membranes
- Multifetal pregnancy

EXPECTED FINDINGS

- Sudden onset of intense localized uterine pain with dark red vaginal bleeding
- Area of uterine tenderness can be localized or diffuse over uterus and boardlike
- Contractions with hypertonicity
- Fetal distress
- Manifestations of hypovolemic shock

LABORATORY TESTS

- Hgb and Hct decreased
- Coagulation factors decreased
- Clotting defects (disseminated intravascular coagulation)
- Cross and type match for possible blood transfusions
- Kleihauer–Betke test (used to detect fetal blood in maternal circulation)

DIAGNOSTIC PROCEDURES

- Ultrasound for fetal well–being and assessment of placenta
- Biophysical profile to ascertain fetal well–being

PATIENT-CENTERED CARE

NURSING CARE

- Palpate the uterus for tenderness and tone.
- Perform serial monitoring of the fundal height.
- Monitor FHR pattern.
- Immediate birth is the management.
  - Administer medications. Monitor IV fluids and blood products.
  - Administer oxygen 8 to 10 L/min via face mask.
  - Monitor maternal vital signs, observing for declining hemodynamic status.
  - Determine urinary output, and monitor fluid balance.

CLIENT EDUCATION

Provide emotional support for the client and family.

Application Exercises

1. A nurse in the emergency department is caring for a client who reports abrupt, sharp, right lower quadrant abdominal pain and bright red vaginal bleeding. The client states she missed one menstrual cycle and cannot be pregnant because she has an intrauterine device. The nurse should suspect which of the following?

   A. Missed abortion

   B. Ectopic pregnancy

   C. Severe preeclampsia

   D. Hydatidiform mole

2. A nurse is assisting with the care for a client who has a marginal abruptio placentae. Which of the following findings are risk factors for developing the condition? (Select all that apply.)

   A. Fetal position

   B. Blunt abdominal trauma

   C. Cocaine use

   D. Maternal age

   E. Cigarette smoking

3. A nurse is assisting with the care for a client who is at 32 weeks of gestation and has a placenta previa. The nurse notes that the client is actively bleeding. Which of the following medications should the nurse anticipate the provider will prescribe?

   A. Betamethasone

   B. Indomethacin

   C. Nifedipine

   D. Methylergonovine

4. A nurse at an antepartum clinic is caring for a client who is at 16 weeks of gestation. The client reports continued nausea and vomiting and scant, prune-colored discharge. She has experienced no weight loss and has a fundal height larger than expected. Which of the following complications should the nurse suspect?

   A. Hyperemesis gravidarum

   B. Threatened abortion

   C. Hydatidiform mole

   D. Preterm labor

5. A nurse is assisting with the care of a client who has a diagnosis of ruptured ectopic pregnancy. Which of the following findings is expected with this condition?

   A. No alteration in menses

   B. Transvaginal ultrasound indicating a fetus in the uterus

   C. Serum progesterone greater than the expected reference range

   D. Report of severe shoulder pain

PRACTICE Active Learning Scenario

A nurse is presenting an educational program on placenta previa for a group of coworkers. What should the nurse manager include in this presentation? Use the ATI Active Learning Template: System Disorder to complete this item.

ALTERATION IN HEALTH (DIAGNOSIS): Describe the three types.

RISK FACTORS: Identify three.

DIAGNOSTIC PROCEDURES: Describe two.

NURSING CARE: Describe nursing action that is contraindicated.

1. A. A client who experienced a missed abortion would report brownish discharge and no pain.

    B. **CORRECT:** Manifestations of an ectopic pregnancy include unilateral lower quadrant pain with or without bleeding. Use of an IUD is a risk factor associated with this condition.

    C. A client who has severe preeclampsia does not have vaginal bleeding and presents with right upper quadrant epigastric pain.

    D. A client who has a hydatidiform mole usually has dark brown vaginal bleeding in the second trimester that is not accompanied by abdominal pain.

    Ⓝ *NCLEX® Connection: Reduction of Risk Potential, Potential for Alterations in Body Systems*

2. A. Fetal position is not a risk factor associated with abruptio placentae.

    B. **CORRECT:** Blunt abdominal trauma is a risk factor associated with abruptio placentae.

    C. **CORRECT:** Cocaine use is a risk factor associated with abruptio placentae.

    D. Maternal age is not a risk factor associated with abruptio placentae.

    E. **CORRECT:** Cigarette smoking is a risk factor associated with abruptio placentae.

    Ⓝ *NCLEX® Connection: Physiological Adaptation, Unexpected Response to Therapies*

3. A. **CORRECT:** Betamethasone is given to promote lung maturity if delivery is anticipated.

    B. Indomethacin is prescribed for the client in preterm labor.

    C. Nifedipine is prescribed for the client in preterm labor.

    D. Methylergonovine is prescribed for the client experiencing postpartum hemorrhage.

    Ⓝ *NCLEX® Connection: Pharmacological Therapies, Medication Administration*

4. A. A client who has hyperemesis gravidarum will have weight loss and manifestations of dehydration.

    B. A client who has a threatened abortion would be in the first trimester and report spotting to moderate bleeding with no enlarged uterus.

    C. **CORRECT:** A client who has a hydatidiform mole exhibits increased fundal height that is inconsistent with the week of gestation, and excessive nausea and vomiting due to elevated hCG levels. Scant, dark discharge occurs in the second trimester.

    D. Preterm labor presents prior to 37 weeks of gestation and is accompanied by pink-stained vaginal discharge and uterine contractions that become more regular.

    Ⓝ *NCLEX® Connection: Reduction of Risk Potential, Potential for Alterations in Body Systems*

5. A. A client experiencing a ruptured ectopic pregnancy has delayed, scant, or irregular menses.

    B. A transvaginal ultrasound would indicate an empty uterus in a client who has a ruptured ectopic pregnancy.

    C. A serum progesterone level lower than the expected reference range is an indication of ectopic pregnancy.

    D. **CORRECT:** A client's report of severe shoulder pain is a manifestation associated with a ruptured ectopic pregnancy due to the presence of blood in the abdominal cavity, which irritates the diaphragm and phrenic nerve.

    Ⓝ *NCLEX® Connection: Reduction of Risk Potential, Potential for Alterations in Body Systems*

PRACTICE Answer

Using the ATI Active Learning Template: System Disorder

ALTERATION IN HEALTH (DIAGNOSIS)
- Complete or total: Cervical os is covered by the placenta.
- Incomplete or partial: Cervical os is only partially covered by the placenta.
- Marginal or low-lying: Placenta is attached in the lower uterine segment but does not reach the cervical os.

RISK FACTORS
- Previous placenta previa
- Uterine scarring due to previous cesarean birth, curettage, or endometritis
- Maternal age 35 to 40 years
- Multifetal gestation
- Multiple gestations or closely spaced pregnancies
- Cigarette smoking

DIAGNOSTIC PROCEDURES
- Transabdominal or transvaginal ultrasound
- Fetal monitoring

NURSING CARE: Performing a vaginal exam

Ⓝ *NCLEX® Connection: Physiological Adaptation, Alterations in Body Systems*

UNIT 1   ANTEPARTUM NURSING CARE
SECTION: COMPLICATIONS OF PREGNANCY

CHAPTER 7 *Infections*

Maternal infections during pregnancy require prompt identification and treatment by a provider. These include human immunodeficiency virus (HIV), acquired immune deficiency syndrome (AIDS), TORCH infections, group B streptococcus (GBS), chlamydia, gonorrhea, syphilis, human papilloma virus (HPV), trichomoniasis, bacterial vaginosis (BV), and candidiasis.

HIV/AIDS

HIV is a retrovirus that attacks and causes destruction of T lymphocytes. It causes immunosuppression in a client. HIV is transmitted from the mother to a neonate perinatally through the placenta and postnatally through breast milk.

- All pregnant clients should be offered testing for HIV as part of routine prenatal testing. Early identification and treatment significantly decreases the incidence of perinatal transmission.
- Testing is recommended in the third trimester for clients who are at an increased risk. Rapid HIV testing should be done if a client is in labor and her HIV status is unknown.

FOR CLIENTS WHO TEST POSITIVE FOR HIV
- Procedures such as amniocentesis and episiotomy should be avoided due to the risk of maternal blood exposure.
- Use of internal fetal monitors, vacuum extraction, and forceps during labor should be avoided due to the risk of fetal bleeding. Qs
- Administration of injections and blood testing in the newborn should not take place until the first bath is given.

DATA COLLECTION

RISK FACTORS
- IV drug use
- Multiple sexual partners
- High-risk sexual partners
- Maternal history of multiple STIs
- Blood transfusion (rare occurrence)

EXPECTED FINDINGS
Fatigue and influenza-like manifestations

PHYSICAL FINDINGS
- Fever
- Diarrhea and weight loss
- Lymphadenopathy and rash
- Anemia

LABORATORY TESTS
- Obtain maternal informed consent prior to testing.
- Testing begins with an antibody screening test, such as enzyme immunoassay. Confirmation of positive results is confirmed by Western blot test or immunofluorescence assay.
- Use rapid HIV antibody test (blood or urine sample) for a client in labor.
- Screen clients for STIs (gonorrhea, chlamydia, syphilis, hepatitis B).
- Obtain frequent viral load levels and CD4 cell counts throughout pregnancy.

PATIENT-CENTERED CARE

NURSING CARE
- Offer counseling prior to and after testing.
- Refer the client for mental health consultation, legal assistance, and financial resources.
- Use standard precautions.
- Administer antiviral prophylaxis, triple drug antiretroviral, or highly active antiretroviral therapy.
- Obtain prescribed laboratory testing.
- Encourage immunization against hepatitis B, pneumococcal infection, *Haemophilus influenzae* type B, and influenza.
  - Recommendations for immunizations change periodically. Check the CDC website (www.cdc.gov) for the most up-to-date recommendations.
- Encourage use of condoms to minimize exposure if a partner is the source of infection.
- Review plan for scheduled cesarean birth at 38 weeks for maternal viral load of more than 1,000 copies/mL.
- Infant should be bathed after birth before remaining with the mother.

MEDICATIONS

Zidovudine

- Antiretroviral agent
- Nucleoside reverse transcriptase inhibitor

NURSING ACTIONS

- Administer zidovudine at 14 weeks of gestation, throughout pregnancy, and before onset of labor or cesarean birth.
- Administer zidovudine to the infant at delivery and for 6 weeks following birth.

REINFORCE CLIENT EDUCATION

DISCHARGE INSTRUCTIONS Qpcc

- Instruct the client not to breastfeed.
- Discuss HIV and safe sexual relations with the client.
- Refer the client and infant to providers specializing in care of clients who have HIV.
- All states have a reportable diseases list. HIV/AIDS is a commonly reported condition. It is the responsibility of the provider to report cases of these diseases to their local health department.

TORCH infections

Toxoplasmosis, other infections (hepatitis), rubella virus, cytomegalovirus, and herpes simplex virus are known collectively as TORCH, which is a group of infections that can negatively affect a client who is pregnant. These infections can cross the placenta and have teratogenic effects on the fetus. TORCH does not include all the major infections that present risks to the mother and fetus.

DATA COLLECTION

RISK FACTORS

- Toxoplasmosis is caused by consumption of raw or undercooked meat or handling cat feces. Manifestations are similar to influenza and lymphadenopathy.
- Other infections include hepatitis A and B, syphilis, mumps, parvovirus B19, and varicella-zoster. These are some of the most common and can be associated with congenital anomalies.
- Rubella (German measles) is contracted through children who have rashes or neonates who are born to women who had rubella during pregnancy.
- Cytomegalovirus (member of herpes virus family) is transmitted by droplet infection from person to person, semen, cervical and vaginal secretions, breast milk, placental tissue, urine, feces, and blood. Latent virus can be reactivated and cause disease to the fetus in utero or during passage through the birth canal.
- Herpes simplex virus (HSV) is spread by direct contact with oral or genital lesions. Transmission to the fetus is greatest during vaginal birth if the woman has active lesions.

EXPECTED FINDINGS

Toxoplasmosis: manifestations similar to influenza or lymphadenopathy (malaise, muscle aches flu-like manifestations)

Rubella: manifestations of joint and muscle pain

Cytomegalovirus: asymptomatic or mononucleosis-like manifestations

Herpes simplex infection: manifestations consisting of painful blisters and tender lymph nodes

PHYSICAL FINDINGS

- Manifestations of toxoplasmosis include fever and tender lymph nodes.
- Manifestations of rubella include rash, mild lymphedema, fever, and fetal consequences, which include miscarriage, congenital anomalies, and death.
- HSV initially presents with lesions and tender lymph nodes. Fetal consequences include miscarriage, preterm labor, and intrauterine growth restriction. A cesarean section is recommended for all clients in labor who have active genital herpes lesions or early manifestations of impending outbreak, such as vulvar pain and itching.

LABORATORY TESTS

For herpes simplex, obtain cultures from clients who have HSV or are at or near term.

DIAGNOSTIC PROCEDURES

- TORCH screen: immunologic survey used to identify existence of these infections in the mother (to identify fetal risks) or newborn (detection of antibodies against infections)
- Prenatal screenings

PATIENT-CENTERED CARE

NURSING CARE

- Monitor fetal well-being.
- Rubella immunization is contraindicated in pregnant women because it is a live virus and rubella infection can develop. These women should avoid crowds of young children. Women who have low titers prior to pregnancy should receive immunizations after giving birth.

MEDICATIONS

- Administer antibiotics.
- Treatment of toxoplasmosis includes sulfonamides or a combination of pyrimethamine and sulfadiazine (potentially harmful to the fetus, but parasitic treatment is essential).

CLIENT EDUCATION Q PCC

- Prevention practices include correct hand hygiene and cooking meat properly. Avoid contact with contaminated cat litter.
- Because no treatment for cytomegalovirus exists, prevent exposure by frequent hand hygiene before eating, and after handling infant diapers and toys.
- Comply with the prescribed treatment.
- Have safe sexual relations.
- Provide emotional support.

Group B streptococcus

GBS is a bacterial infection that can be passed to a fetus during labor and delivery. All pregnant clients are screened for GBS during the third trimester.

DATA COLLECTION

EXPECTED FINDINGS

PHYSICAL FINDINGS: Positive GBS can have maternal and fetal effects.

- Premature rupture of membranes
- Preterm labor and delivery
- Chorioamnionitis
- Infections of the urinary tract
- Maternal sepsis

LABORATORY TESTS

Vaginal and rectal cultures are performed at 35 to 37 weeks of gestation.

PATIENT-CENTERED CARE

NURSING CARE

Administer intrapartum antibiotic prophylaxis to the following clients.

- Client who has GBS bacteriuria during current pregnancy
- Client who has a GBS–positive screening during current pregnancy
- Client who has unknown GBS status who is delivering at less than 37 weeks of gestation

MEDICATIONS

- Bactericidal antibiotic is used to destroy the GBS.
- Penicillin G or ampicillin are most commonly prescribed for GBS.
- Ask the charge nurse to administer penicillin 5 million units IV as a loading dose, followed by 2.5 million units via intermittent IV bolus every 4 hr until delivery. The client can receive ampicillin 2 g IV initially, followed by 1 g every 4 hr via intermittent IV bolus.

CLIENT EDUCATION

Notify the labor and delivery nurse of GBS status.

Chlamydia

Chlamydia is a bacterial infection caused by *Chlamydia trachomatis* and is the most commonly reported STI in American women.

- The infection can be difficult to diagnose because it is often asymptomatic. If chlamydia is left untreated in women, it can lead to pelvic inflammatory disease (PID), which can cause infertility.
- The Centers for Disease Control and Prevention (CDC) recommends yearly screening of all sexually active women younger than 25 years, as well as older women who have risk factors (new or multiple partners). All pregnant clients should be screened at the first prenatal visit and rescreened in the third trimester if younger than 25 years or at high risk.

DATA COLLECTION

RISK FACTORS

- Multiple sexual partners
- Unprotected sex

EXPECTED FINDINGS

Male clients

- Urethral discharge
- Dysuria

PHYSICAL FINDINGS: Mucoid or watery urethral discharge

Female clients

- Dysuria
- Urinary frequency
- Spotting or postcoital bleeding

PHYSICAL FINDINGS
- Mucopurulent endocervical discharge
- Easily induced endocervical bleeding

LABORATORY TESTS

- Urine culture preferred for male clients
- Endocervical culture preferred for female clients

PATIENT-CENTERED CARE

NURSING CARE

- Identify and treat all sexual partners.
- Clients who are pregnant should be retested 3 weeks after completing the prescribed regimen.

MEDICATIONS

Azithromycin or amoxicillin

- Prescribed during pregnancy
- Broad-spectrum antibiotic
- Bactericidal action

NURSING ACTIONS: Administer erythromycin eye ointment to all infants following delivery. This is the medication of choice for ophthalmia neonatorum. This antibiotic is both bacteriostatic and bactericidal, and thus provides prophylaxis against *Neisseria gonorrhoeae* and *Chlamydia trachomatis*.

CLIENT EDUCATION

- Take all medication as prescribed.
- There is a possibility of decreasing effectiveness of oral contraceptives. Qpcc
- Safe sex practices include mutual monogamy and correct, consistent condom use.
- All states have a reportable diseases list. Chlamydia is a commonly reported condition. It is the responsibility of the provider to report cases of these diseases to the local health department.

Gonorrhea

Neisseria gonorrhoeae is the causative agent of gonorrhea. Gonorrhea is a bacterial infection that is primarily spread by genital-to-genital contact. However, it also can be spread by anal-to-genital or oral-to-genital contact. It can also be transmitted to a newborn during delivery.

- Women are frequently asymptomatic. Untreated gonorrhea can lead to PID, which can cause infertility.
- The CDC recommends yearly screening for all sexually active women younger than 25 years as well as older women who have risk factors (new or multiple sex partners). All pregnant women should be screened at the first prenatal visit and rescreened in the third trimester if at high risk.

DATA COLLECTION

RISK FACTORS

- Multiple sexual partners
- Unprotected sexual practices

EXPECTED FINDINGS

Male clients

- Dysuria
- Urethral discharge

Female clients

- Dysuria
- Vaginal bleeding between periods and dysmenorrhea

PHYSICAL FINDINGS
- Yellowish-green vaginal discharge
- Easily induced endocervical bleeding

LABORATORY TESTS

- Urine culture preferred for male clients
- Endocervical culture preferred for female clients

PATIENT-CENTERED CARE

NURSING CARE

- Identify and treat all sexual partners.
- Administer erythromycin eye ointment to all infants following delivery. This is the medication of choice for ophthalmia neonatorum. This antibiotic is both bacteriostatic and bactericidal, and thus provides prophylaxis against *Neisseria gonorrhoeae* and *Chlamydia trachomatis*.

MEDICATIONS

Ceftriaxone IM and azithromycin PO: Broad-spectrum antibiotic; bactericidal action

CLIENT EDUCATION

- Disease transmission.
- Take all medications as prescribed.
- Repeat the culture to evaluate for medication effectiveness.
- There is a possibility of decreasing effectiveness of oral contraceptives.
- Safe sex practices include mutual monogamy and correct, consistent condom use.
- All states have a reportable diseases list. Gonorrhea is a commonly reported condition. It is the responsibility of the provider to report cases of these diseases to the local health department.

Syphilis

Syphilis is an STI caused by the bacterium *Treponema pallidum*. It can have long-term complications if not adequately treated.

- Syphilis has three stages.
  - **Primary:** Characterized by presence of a chancre
  - **Secondary:** Characterized by skin rashes, such as a rash on the palms of hands and soles of feet
  - **Tertiary:** Characterized by damage to internal organs
- Black, Hispanic, and other racial/ethnic minority groups are disproportionately affected by syphilis in the U.S.
- It can be transmitted through oral, vaginal, or anal sex, as well as transmitted to an unborn child. Though the rate of congenital syphilis has recently decreased, more cases of congenital syphilis are reported in the U.S. than cases of perinatal HIV infection.
- All pregnant clients should be screened at the first prenatal visit and rescreened in the third trimester if at high risk (live in areas with high numbers of syphilis cases; not previously tested; had positive test in the first trimester).

DATA COLLECTION

RISK FACTORS

- Multiple partners
- Unprotected sexual practices

EXPECTED FINDINGS

Primary stage: A chancre or sore in the genital area.

Secondary stage: Skin rashes, such as a rash on the palmar surface of the hands and the soles of the feet.

Tertiary stage: Damage to internal organs can occur for which clients can notice the manifestations including difficulty coordinating muscle movements and blindness.

LABORATORY TESTS

Serology tests: Nontreponemal (VDRL and rapid plasma reagin) and treponemal (enzyme immunoassay, immunoassays)

- Nontreponemal tests are often used for screening then treponemal tests to detect antibodies specific for syphilis to confirm the diagnosis.
- This sequence of nontreponemal then treponemal tests is considered the standard for testing.

PATIENT-CENTERED CARE

MEDICATIONS

Penicillin G IM in a single dose

CLIENT EDUCATION

- Abstain from sexual contact until sores have completely healed.
- Partners need to be tested and treated.
- Safe sex practices include mutual monogamy and correct, consistent condom use.
- All states have a reportable diseases list. Syphilis is a commonly reported condition. It is the responsibility of the provider to report cases of these diseases to the local health department.

Human papilloma virus

HPV is the most common viral STI. Some types can cause genital warts (also known as *Condyloma acuminata*) and cancers.

- It is spread through oral, vaginal, and anal sex (most commonly vaginal or anal routes). When large, widespread, or occluding the birth canal, genital warts can complicate a vaginal delivery. Therefore, a cesarean section can be recommended.
- Routine screening for women 21 to 65 years old can provide early detection. Screening should occur even during pregnancy.

DATA COLLECTION

RISK FACTORS

- Multiple partners
- Unprotected sexual practices

EXPECTED FINDINGS

Client reports painless bumps in the genital area.

PHYSICAL FINDINGS

- Small warts or a group of warts in the genital area that can have a cauliflower-like appearance
- Abnormal changes to the cervix that can be detected by a Pap test

LABORATORY TESTS

Pap test with or without HPV co-testing per American Cancer Society and American Congress of Obstetricians and Gynecologists guidelines.

- Women 21 to 29 years old should have a Pap test every 3 years.
- Women 30 to 65 years old should have both a Pap test and an HPV test every 5 years (preferred). It is also acceptable to have a Pap test every 3 years.
- Women older than 65 years who have had regular screenings with normal results should not be screened for cervical cancer, unless they have cervical precancer, in which they should continue to be screened for 20 years after the precancer diagnosis.

DIAGNOSTIC PROCEDURES

- Genital warts are diagnosed by the provider based on appearance.
- Based on the Pap test result, colposcopy and biopsy can be performed to diagnose cervical precancer and cancer.

PATIENT-CENTERED CARE

MEDICATIONS

For genital warts and *Condyloma acuminata,* options include a client-applied cream, such as imiquimod, if not pregnant or a provider-administered therapy (cryotherapy, trichloroacetic acid application).

THERAPEUTIC PROCEDURES

For precancerous changes on the cervix, the provider can perform treatments including laser therapy or cone biopsy. For a pregnant client who has an abnormal Pap that requires further follow-up, further evaluation and treatment are usually deferred until after birth.

CLIENT EDUCATION

- Vaccines are recommended to protect against low-risk types of HPV that cause genital warts and high-risk types of HPV that cause cancer. The vaccine is recommended for clients 9 to 26 years of age, though ideally given at age 11 to 12 years.
- Safe sex practices include mutual monogamy and correct, consistent condom use.

Trichomoniasis

Trichomoniasis is an STI caused by the protozoan parasite *Trichomonas vaginalis.* It can be spread through genital-to-genital contact.

- If trichomoniasis is left untreated in women, it can lead to PID, which can cause infertility. All women who have manifestations should be tested.
- Pregnant clients who have trichomoniasis are more likely to have preterm delivery and babies with low birth weight (less than 5.5 lb).

DATA COLLECTION

RISK FACTORS

- Multiple partners
- Unprotected sexual practices

EXPECTED FINDINGS

Male clients

- Penile itching or irritation
- Dysuria

PHYSICAL FINDINGS: Urethral discharge, which can be swabbed for microscopy

Female clients

- Yellow-green, frothy vaginal discharge with foul odor
- Dyspareunia and itching
- Dysuria

PHYSICAL FINDINGS
- Discharge in the vaginal vault, which can be sampled for microscopy
- Strawberry spots on the cervix (tiny petechiae)
- A cervix that bleeds easily

LABORATORY TESTS

A sample of the discharge is used for application to pH paper and wet mount.

DIAGNOSTIC PROCEDURES

- pH greater than 4.5
- Wet mount saline prep indicates the presence of trichomonad(s).

PATIENT-CENTERED CARE

MEDICATIONS

Anti-infective: Metronidazole or tinidazole orally in a single dose

CLIENT EDUCATION

- Avoid alcohol while taking this medication due to the disulfiram-like reaction that occurs (severe nausea and vomiting).
- Take all medication as prescribed.
- There is a possibility of decreasing effectiveness of oral contraceptives.
- Identify and treat all sexual partners.
- Safe sex practices include mutual monogamy and correct, consistent condom use.

Bacterial vaginosis

A bacterial infection most commonly caused by *Haemophilus vaginalis* or *Gardnerella vaginalis*, it is the most common vaginal infection in women 15 to 44 years old. It is not considered an STI, but having multiple sex partners can increase the risk.

- If BV is left untreated, it can increase a woman's chances of developing PID, which can lead to infertility. All women who have manifestations should be tested.
- Treatment is especially important for pregnant clients. BV is associated with preterm labor and babies with low birth weight (less than 5.5 lb).

DATA COLLECTION

RISK FACTORS

- New or multiple sex partners
- Unprotected sexual practices
- Altered pH balance of vagina, such as caused by douching

EXPECTED FINDINGS

Thin, white or gray discharge with a fish-like odor, especially after sex

PHYSICAL FINDINGS: Discharge in the vaginal vault, which can be sampled for microscopy

LABORATORY TESTS

- Sample of the discharge used for application to pH paper
- Wet mount and whiff test performed

DIAGNOSTIC PROCEDURES

- pH greater than 4.5
- Wet mount saline prep indicates presence of clue cells.
- Positive whiff test

PATIENT-CENTERED CARE

MEDICATIONS

Metronidazole: Anti-infective

CLIENT EDUCATION

- Avoid alcohol while taking this medication due to a disulfiram-like reaction (severe nausea and vomiting).
- Take all medications as prescribed.
- There is a possibility of decreasing effectiveness of oral contraceptives.
- Treatment is not usually indicated for male partners.
- Safe sex practices include mutual monogamy and correct, consistent condom use.
- Avoid tight-fitting clothing.
- Wear cotton-lined underpants.
- Avoid douching.

Candidiasis

Candidiasis, also known as vulvovaginal candidiasis or yeast infection, is a fungal infection caused by *Candida albicans*.

- It is the second most common type of vaginal infection in the U.S.
- All women who have manifestations should be tested.

DATA COLLECTION

RISK FACTORS

- Pregnancy
- Diabetes mellitus
- Oral contraceptive use
- Recent antibiotic treatment
- Obesity
- Diet high in refined sugars

EXPECTED FINDINGS

Vulvar and vaginal pruritus

PHYSICAL FINDINGS

- Thick, creamy, white, cottage cheese–like vaginal discharge
- Vulvar and vaginal erythema and inflammation
- White patches on vaginal walls
- Gray-white patches on the tongue and gums (neonate)

LABORATORY TESTS

- Sample of discharge used for application to pH paper
- Wet mount and whiff test performed

DIAGNOSTIC PROCEDURES

- pH less than 4.5 (normal pH)
- Wet mount potassium hydroxide prep indicates presence of yeast buds, hyphae, and pseudohyphae.
- Negative whiff test

PATIENT-CENTERED CARE

MEDICATIONS

Oral fluconazole

- Antifungal agent
- Can be prescribed as a single low dose
- Topical therapies recommended for use in pregnant clients

Over-the-counter treatments

OTC treatments, such as clotrimazole, are available to treat candidiasis. However, it is important for the provider to diagnose candidiasis initially.

CLIENT EDUCATION

- Avoid tight-fitting clothing.
- Wear cotton-lined underpants.
- Limit wearing damp clothing.
- Avoid douching.

Application Exercises

1. A nurse is admitting a client who is in labor and has an HIV infection HIV. The nurse should identify that HIV infection is a contraindication to which of the following interventions? (Select all that apply.)
   - A. Episiotomy
   - B. Oxytocin infusion
   - C. Forceps
   - D. Cesarean birth
   - E. Internal fetal monitoring

2. A nurse in an antepartum clinic is collecting data on a client who has a TORCH infection. Which of the following findings should the nurse expect? (Select all that apply.)
   - A. Joint pain
   - B. Malaise
   - C. Rash
   - D. Urinary frequency
   - E. Tender lymph nodes

3. A nurse is caring for a client who has gonorrhea. Which of the following medications should the nurse anticipate the provider will prescribe?
   - A. Ceftriaxone
   - B. Fluconazole
   - C. Metronidazole
   - D. Zidovudine

4. A nurse is caring for a client who is in labor. The nurse should identify that which of the following infections can be treated during labor or immediately following birth? (Select all that apply.)
   - A. Gonorrhea
   - B. Chlamydia
   - C. HIV
   - D. Group B streptococcus beta-hemolytic
   - E. TORCH infection

5. A nurse manager is reviewing ways to prevent a TORCH infection during pregnancy with a group of newly licensed nurses. Which of the following statements by a nurse indicates understanding of the teaching?
   - A. "Obtain an immunization against rubella early in pregnancy."
   - B. "Seek prophylactic treatment if cytomegalovirus is detected during pregnancy."
   - C. "A woman should avoid crowded places during pregnancy."
   - D. "A woman should avoid consuming undercooked meat while pregnant."

PRACTICE Active Learning Scenario

A nurse is planning care for a client who is pregnant and positive for group B streptococcus beta-hemolytic. Use the ATI Active Learning Template: System Disorder to complete this item.

LABORATORY TESTS: Describe the test and when it is performed.

RISK FACTORS: Describe two maternal risk factors and three fetal risk factors.

MEDICATIONS: Describe three clients who should receive intrapartum antibiotic prophylaxis.

Application Exercises Key

1. A. **CORRECT:** An episiotomy should be avoided for a client who is HIV-positive due to the risk of maternal blood exposure.

   B. Oxytocin infusion is not contraindicated for this client.

   C. **CORRECT:** The use of forceps during delivery should be avoided due to the risk of fetal and maternal bleeding.

   D. Cesarean birth is not contraindicated for this client.

   E. **CORRECT:** Internal fetal monitoring should be avoided due to the risk of fetal bleeding.

   Ⓝ *NCLEX® Connection: Reduction of Risk Potential, Potential for Complications of Diagnostic Tests/Treatments/Procedures*

2. A. **CORRECT:** TORCH infections are flu-like in presentation, such as joint pain.

   B. **CORRECT:** TORCH infections are flu-like in presentation, such as malaise.

   C. **CORRECT:** TORCH infections can include findings such as a rash.

   D. Urinary frequency is not a manifestation associated with a TORCH infection.

   E. **CORRECT:** TORCH infections are flu-like in presentation, such as tender lymph nodes.

   Ⓝ *NCLEX® Connection: Physiological Adaptation, Alterations in Body Systems*

3. A. **CORRECT:** Ceftriaxone IM or doxycycline orally for 7 days is prescribed for the treatment of gonorrhea.

   B. Fluconazole is used to treat candidiasis.

   C. Metronidazole is used in the treatment of bacterial vaginosis and trichomoniasis.

   D. Zidovudine is used to treat HIV/AIDS.

   Ⓝ *NCLEX® Connection: Pharmacological Therapies, Expected Actions/Outcomes*

4. A. **CORRECT:** Erythromycin is administered to the infant immediately following delivery to prevent *Neisseria gonorrhoeae*.

   B. **CORRECT:** Erythromycin is administered to the infant immediately following delivery to prevent *Chlamydia trachomatis*.

   C. **CORRECT:** Zidovudine is prescribed to a client in labor who is HIV-positive.

   D. **CORRECT:** Penicillin G or ampicillin may be prescribed to treat positive GBS.

   E. A TORCH infection can be treated during pregnancy depending upon the infection.

   Ⓝ *NCLEX® Connection: Physiological Adaptation, Alterations in Body Systems*

5. A. Immunization against rubella is contraindicated during pregnancy due to the risk of fetal congenital anomalies.

   B. There is no treatment for cytomegalovirus.

   C. A TORCH infection cannot be transmitted by being in areas where large crowds are present.

   D. **CORRECT:** Toxoplasmosis, a TORCH infection, is contracted by consuming undercooked meat.

   Ⓝ *NCLEX® Connection: Physiological Adaptation, Alterations in Body Systems*

PRACTICE Answer

Using the ATI Active Learning Template: System Disorder

LABORATORY TESTS: Vaginal and rectal cultures performed at 35 to 37 weeks of gestation

RISK FACTORS
- Maternal
  - History of positive culture with previous pregnancy
  - Maternal age less than 20 years
  - African American or Hispanic ethnicity
- Fetal
  - Positive during pregnancy
  - Prolonged rupture of membranes
  - Preterm delivery
  - Low birth weight
  - Use of intrauterine fetal monitoring
  - Intrapartum maternal fever (38° C [100.4° F])

MEDICATIONS
- Client who has GBS bacteriuria during current pregnancy
- Client who has a GBS-positive screen during current pregnancy
- Client who has unknown GBS status who is delivering at less than 37 weeks of gestation
- Client who has maternal fever of 38° C (100.4° F)
- Client who has rupture of membranes for 18 hr or longer

Ⓝ *NCLEX® Connection: Reduction of Risk Potential, Potential for Alterations in Body Systems*

UNIT 1   ANTEPARTUM NURSING CARE
SECTION: COMPLICATIONS OF PREGNANCY

CHAPTER 8 *Medical Conditions*

Unexpected medical conditions can occur during pregnancy. Awareness, early detection, and interventions are crucial components to ensure fetal well-being and maternal health.

Unexpected medical conditions include cervical insufficiency, hyperemesis gravidarum, anemia, gestational diabetes mellitus (GDM), and gestational hypertension (GH).

Cervical insufficiency (premature cervical dilatation)

Cervical insufficiency is a condition whereby the cervix opens too early and expulsion of the products of conception occurs. It is thought to be related to tissue changes and alterations in the length of the cervix.

DATA COLLECTION

RISK FACTORS

- History of cervical trauma (cervical tears from previous deliveries, excessive dilations, curettage for biopsy, surgical procedures involving the cervix), short labors, pregnancy loss in early gestation, or advanced cervical dilation at earlier weeks of gestation
- In utero exposure to diethylstilbestrol, ingested by the client's mother during pregnancy
- Congenital structural defects of the uterus or cervix

EXPECTED FINDINGS

Increase in pelvic pressure or urge to push

PHYSICAL FINDINGS
- Pink-stained vaginal discharge or bleeding
- Possible gush of fluid (rupture of membranes)
- Uterine contractions with the expulsion of the fetus

DIAGNOSTIC AND THERAPEUTIC PROCEDURES

- An **ultrasound** showing a short cervix (less than 25 mm in length), presence of cervical funneling (beaking), or effacement of the cervical os indicates reduced cervical competence.
- **Prophylactic cervical cerclage** is the surgical reinforcement of the cervix with a suture to strengthen it and prevent premature cervical dilation. Best results occur if this is done at 12 to 14 weeks of gestation. The cerclage is removed between 36 and 38 weeks of gestation or when spontaneous labor occurs.

PATIENT-CENTERED CARE

NURSING CARE

- Evaluate the client's support systems and availability of assistance if activity restrictions or bed rest are prescribed.
- Monitor vaginal discharge.
- Monitor client reports of pressure and contractions.
- Monitor postoperative (cerclage) for uterine contractions, rupture of membranes, and manifestations of infection.

MEDICATIONS

Administer tocolytics prophylactically to inhibit uterine contractions.

CLIENT EDUCATION

DISCHARGE INSTRUCTIONS
- Place the client on activity restriction or bed rest.
- Encourage hydration to promote a relaxed uterus. (Dehydration stimulates uterine contractions.)
- Avoid intercourse, tampons, and douching, and monitor for cervical/uterine changes.

HEALTH PROMOTION AND DISEASE PREVENTION
- Instruct the client about findings to report to the provider (preterm labor, rupture of membranes, infection, strong contractions less than 5 min apart, severe perineal pressure, an urge to push).
- Instruct the client about using the home uterine activity monitor to evaluate uterine contractions.

NURSING ACTIONS
- Arrange for the client to follow up with a home health facility for close observation and supervision.
- Plan for removal of the cerclage between 36 and 38 weeks of gestation.

Hyperemesis gravidarum

- Hyperemesis gravidarum is excessive nausea and vomiting (possibly related to elevated hCG levels) that is prolonged past 12 weeks of gestation and results in a 5% weight loss from prepregnancy weight, electrolyte imbalance, acetonuria, and ketosis.
- There is a risk to the fetus for intrauterine growth restriction or preterm birth if the condition persists.

DATA COLLECTION

RISK FACTORS

- Maternal age younger than 30 years
- Multifetal gestation
- Gestational trophoblastic disease or fetus with chromosomal anomaly
- Psychosocial issues and high levels of emotional stress
- Clinical hyperthyroid disorders
- Diabetes
- Gastrointestinal disorders
- Family history of hyperemesis

EXPECTED FINDINGS

PHYSICAL FINDINGS
- Excessive vomiting for prolonged periods
- Dehydration with possible electrolyte imbalance
- Weight loss
- Increased pulse rate
- Decreased blood pressure
- Poor skin turgor and dry mucous membranes

LABORATORY TESTS

- **Urinalysis** for ketones and acetones (breakdown of protein and fat)
  - The most important laboratory test is positive ketonuria.
  - Elevated urine specific gravity
- **Chemistry profile** reveals electrolyte imbalances.
  - Sodium, potassium, and chloride reduced from low intake
  - Metabolic acidosis (secondary to starvation)
  - Metabolic alkalosis due to excessive vomiting
  - Elevated liver enzymes
  - Bilirubin level
- **Thyroid test** indicates hyperthyroidism.
- **Complete blood count** (CBC): Hct concentration is elevated because inability to retain fluid results in hemoconcentration.

PATIENT-CENTERED CARE

NURSING CARE

- Monitor I&O.
- Evaluate skin turgor and mucous membranes.
- Monitor vital signs.
- Monitor weight.
- Have the client remain NPO for 24 to 48 hr.
- Advance to clear liquids after 24 hr if no vomiting.
- Advance the client's diet as tolerated, with frequent small meals.
- In severe cases, or if vomiting returns, enteral nutrition per feeding tube or total parental nutrition can be considered.

MEDICATIONS

- Administer IV lactated Ringer's for hydration.
- Give pyridoxine (vitamin B_6) and other vitamin supplements as tolerated. The American Congress of Obstetricians and Gynecologists recommend the use of pyridoxine alone or in combination with doxylamine as the initial medication management because these medications are considered both safe and effective.
- Use antiemetic medications (ondansetron, metoclopramide) cautiously for uncontrollable nausea and vomiting.

CLIENT EDUCATION

DISCHARGE INSTRUCTIONS: When beginning diet, start with dry toast, crackers, or cereal; then move to a soft diet; and finally to a regular diet as tolerated. ⓠEBP

Iron-deficiency anemia

Iron-deficiency anemia occurs during pregnancy due to inadequacy in maternal iron stores and consuming insufficient amounts of dietary iron.

DATA COLLECTION

RISK FACTORS

- Less than 2 years between pregnancies
- Heavy menses
- Diet low in iron
- Multifetal gestation
- Vomiting frequently due to morning sickness

EXPECTED FINDINGS

- Fatigue and weakness
- Irritability
- Headache
- Dizziness or lightheadedness
- Shortness of breath with exertion
- Palpitations
- Craving unusual food (pica)

PHYSICAL FINDINGS
- Pallor
- Brittle nails
- Shortness of breath

LABORATORY TESTS

- **Hgb** less than 11 mg/dL in the first and third trimesters and less than 10.5 mg/dL in the second trimester
- **Hct** less than 33%

PATIENT-CENTERED CARE

NURSING CARE

- The recommended iron intake for pregnant clients is 27 mg/day. Prenatal vitamins typically contain 30 mg iron. If maternal iron deficiency anemia is present, increased dosages of 60 to 120 mg/day can be required.
- Increase dietary intake of foods rich in iron (legumes, fruit, green leafy vegetables, meat).
- Reinforce client education about ways to minimize gastrointestinal adverse effects.

MEDICATIONS

Ferrous sulfate iron supplements

CLIENT EDUCATION
- Take the supplement with orange juice on an empty stomach to increase absorption.
- A diet rich in vitamin C-containing foods increases absorption.
- Increase roughage and fluid intake in diet to assist with discomforts of constipation.

Iron dextran IV or IM

Used in the treatment of iron-deficiency anemia when oral iron supplements cannot be tolerated.

Gestational diabetes mellitus

- GDM is an impaired tolerance to glucose with the first onset or recognition during pregnancy. The ideal blood glucose level during pregnancy is 70 to 110 mg/dL.
- Manifestations of diabetes mellitus can disappear a few weeks following delivery. However, approximately 50% of women will develop type 2 diabetes mellitus within 5 years.

INCREASED RISKS TO CLIENT AND FETUS
- **Spontaneous abortion** related to poor glycemic control
- **Infections** (urinary and vaginal) related to increased glucose in the urine and decreased resistance because of altered carbohydrate metabolism
- **Hydramnios**, which can cause overdistention of the uterus, premature rupture of membranes, preterm labor, and hemorrhage
- **Ketoacidosis** from diabetogenic effect of pregnancy (increased insulin resistance), untreated hyperglycemia, or inappropriate insulin dosing
- **Hypoglycemia** caused by overdosing in insulin, skipped or late meals, or increased exercise
- **Hyperglycemia**, which can cause excessive fetal growth (macrosomia)

DATA COLLECTION

RISK FACTORS

- Obesity
- Hypertension
- Glycosuria
- Maternal age older than 25 years
- Family history of diabetes mellitus
- Previous delivery of an infant that was large or stillborn

EXPECTED FINDINGS

Hypoglycemia: nervousness, headache, weakness, irritability, hunger, blurred vision, tingling of mouth or extremities

Hyperglycemia: polydipsia, polyphagia, polyuria, nausea, abdominal pain, flushed dry skin, fruity breath

PHYSICAL FINDINGS
- Hypoglycemia
- Shaking
- Clammy pale skin
- Shallow respirations
- Rapid pulse
- Hyperglycemia
- Vomiting
- Excess weight gain during pregnancy

LABORATORY TESTS

- **Routine urinalysis** with glycosuria
- **1-hr glucose tolerance test:** 50 g oral glucose load, followed by plasma glucose analysis 1 hr later performed at 24 to 28 weeks of gestation; fasting not necessary; a positive blood glucose screening is 130 to 140 mg/dL or greater; additional testing with a 3-hr oral glucose tolerance test (OGTT) is indicated ○EBP
- **Oral glucose tolerance test** following overnight fasting, avoidance of caffeine, and abstinence from smoking for 12 hr prior to testing; a fasting glucose is obtained, a 100 g glucose load is given, and serum glucose levels are determined at 1, 2, and 3 hr following glucose ingestion
- **Presence of ketones in urine** to determine severity of ketoacidosis

DIAGNOSTIC PROCEDURES

- Biophysical profile to ascertain fetal well-being
- Amniocentesis with alpha-fetoprotein
- Nonstress test to determine fetal well-being

PATIENT-CENTERED CARE

NURSING CARE

- Monitor the client's blood glucose.
- Monitor the fetus.

MEDICATIONS

In contrast to type 1 diabetes mellitus, GDM is managed initially with diet and exercise alone. If glucose levels are persistently high, insulin is begun.

Oral hypoglycemic therapy is an alternative to insulin in clients who have GDM and require medication in addition to diet for blood glucose control. Most oral hypoglycemic agents are contraindicated for GDM, but there is limited use of glyburide. The provider makes the determination if these medications can be used.

CLIENT EDUCATION

- Perform daily kick counts.
- Reinforce client education about diet, including standard diabetic diet and restricted carbohydrate intake. Dietary counseling by a registered dietitian should occur.
- Reinforce client education about exercise.
- Instruct the client about self-administration of insulin.
- Reinforce client education about the need for postpartum laboratory testing to include OGTT and blood glucose levels.

Gestational hypertension

- Hypertensive disease in pregnancy is divided into clinical subsets of the disease based on end-organ effects and progresses along a continuum from mild gestational hypertension; preeclampsia; and eclampsia.
- Vasospasm contributing to poor tissue perfusion is the underlying mechanism for the manifestations of pregnancy hypertensive disorders.
- Gestational hypertensive disease and chronic hypertension can occur simultaneously.
- Gestational hypertensive diseases are associated with placental abruption, kidney failure, hepatic rupture, preterm birth, and fetal and maternal death.

Gestational hypertension begins after the 20th week of pregnancy and occurs when a pregnant client has an elevated blood pressure at 140/90 mm Hg or greater recorded on two different occasions, at least 4 hr apart. There is no proteinuria. The presence of edema is no longer considered in the definition of hypertensive disease of pregnancy. Blood pressure returns to baseline by 6 weeks postpartum.

Preeclampsia is GH with the addition of proteinuria. In the absence of proteinuria, the development of new-onset hypertension with the new onset of any of the following: thrombocytopenia, renal insufficiency, impaired liver function, pulmonary edema, or cerebral or visual manifestations. Report of transient headaches might occur along with episodes of irritability.

Severe preeclampsia consists of blood pressure that is 160/110 mm Hg or greater, elevated serum creatinine greater than 1.1 mg/dL, cerebral or visual disturbances (headache and blurred vision), hepatic dysfunction, and thrombocytopenia.

Eclampsia is severe preeclampsia manifestations with the onset of seizure activity or coma. Eclampsia is usually preceded by headache, severe epigastric pain, hyperreflexia, and hemoconcentrations, which are warning signs of probable convulsions.

- HELLP syndrome is a diagnosis based on laboratory findings in which hematologic conditions coexist with severe preeclampsia involving hepatic dysfunction.
- **H: Hemolysis** resulting in anemia and jaundice
- **EL: Elevated liver enzymes** resulting in elevated alanine aminotransferase (ALT) or aspartate transaminase (AST), epigastric pain, nausea, and vomiting
- **LP: Low platelets** (less than 100,000/mm³), resulting in thrombocytopenia, abnormal bleeding and clotting time, bleeding gums, petechiae, and possibly disseminated intravascular coagulopathy

DATA COLLECTION

RISK FACTORS

No single profile identifies risks for gestational hypertensive disorders, but some high risks include the following.
- Maternal age younger than 19 or older than 40 years
- First pregnancy
- Morbid obesity
- Multifetal gestation
- Chronic kidney disease
- Chronic hypertension
- Familiar history of preeclampsia
- Diabetes mellitus
- Rheumatoid arthritis
- Systemic lupus erythematosus

EXPECTED FINDINGS

- Severe continuous headache
- Nausea
- Blurring of vision
- Flashes of lights or dots before the eyes

PHYSICAL FINDINGS
- Hypertension
- Proteinuria
- Periorbital, facial, hand, and abdominal edema
- Pitting edema of lower extremities
- Vomiting
- Oliguria
- Hyperreflexia
- Scotoma
- Epigastric pain
- Right upper quadrant pain
- Dyspnea
- Diminished breath sounds
- Manifestations of progression of hypertensive disease with indications of worsening liver involvement, kidney failure, worsening hypertension, cerebral involvement, and developing coagulopathies

ABNORMAL LABORATORY FINDINGS
- Elevated liver enzymes (LDH, AST)
- Increased creatinine
- Increased plasma uric acid
- Thrombocytopenia
- Decreased Hgb
- Hyperbilirubinemia

LABORATORY TESTS

- Liver enzymes
- Serum creatinine, BUN, uric acid, and magnesium increase as renal function decreases
- CBC
- Clotting studies
- Chemistry profile

DIAGNOSTIC PROCEDURES

- 24-hr urine collection for protein and creatinine clearance
- Nonstress test, biophysical profile, and serial ultrasounds to determine fetal status

PATIENT-CENTERED CARE

NURSING CARE

- Monitor level of consciousness.
- Obtain pulse oximetry.
- Monitor I&O.
- Obtain daily weights.
- Monitor vital signs with careful attention to blood pressure measurement (using proper size cuff, avoiding talking to client during measurement).
- Encourage lateral positioning.
- Perform NST and daily kick counts.
- Monitor deep tendon reflexes.

MEDICATIONS

It is recommended that daily low-dose aspirin therapy be initiated late in the first trimester for women who have a history of early onset preeclampsia.

Antihypertensive medications

Methyldopa, nifedipine, hydralazine, labetalol
Avoid ACE inhibitors and angiotensin II receptor blockers.

Anticonvulsant medications

Magnesium sulfate: Medication of choice to depress the CNS and prevent seizures.

NURSING ACTIONS
- Use an infusion control device to maintain a regular flow rate.
- Inform the client that she can initially feel flushed, hot, and sedated with the magnesium sulfate bolus.
- Monitor blood pressure, heart rate, respiratory rate, deep tendon reflexes, level of consciousness, urinary output (indwelling urinary catheter for accuracy), presence of headache, visual disturbances, epigastric pain, uterine contractions, and fetal heart rate and activity.

- Place the client on fluid restriction of 100 to 125 mL/hr, and maintain a urinary output of 30 mL/hr or greater.
- Monitor for manifestations of magnesium sulfate toxicity. Qs
  - Absence of patellar deep tendon reflexes
  - Urine output less than 30 mL/hr
  - Respirations less than 12/min
  - Decreased level of consciousness
  - Cardiac dysrhythmias
- If magnesium toxicity is suspected
  - Immediately discontinue infusion.
  - Administer antidote calcium gluconate or calcium chloride. Qs
  - Prepare for actions to prevent respiratory or cardiac arrest.

CLIENT EDUCATION

DISCHARGE INSTRUCTIONS
- Maintain bed rest and encourage side-lying position.
- Promote diversional activities (TV, visits from family or friends, gentle exercise).
- Avoid foods that are high in sodium.
- Avoid alcohol and tobacco, and limit caffeine intake.
- Drink six to eight 8-oz glasses of water per day.
- Maintain a dark, quiet environment to avoid stimuli that can precipitate a seizure.
- Maintain a patent airway in the event of a seizure.
- Administer antihypertensive medications as prescribed.

Application Exercises

1. A nurse is caring for a client who is at 14 weeks of gestation and has hyperemesis gravidarum. The nurse should identify that which of the following are risk factors for the client? (Select all that apply.)

   A. Obesity

   B. Multifetal pregnancy

   C. Maternal age greater than 40

   D. Migraine headache

   E. Oligohydramnios

2. A nurse is reviewing laboratory results for a client who has suspected hyperemesis gravidarum. Which of the following results should the nurse identify as a manifestation of this condition?

   A. Hgb 12.2 g/dL

   B. Urine ketones present

   C. Alanine aminotransferase 20 IU/L

   D. Serum glucose 114 mg/dL

3. A nurse is assisting in the care of a client who has severe preeclampsia and is receiving magnesium sulfate via continuous IV infusion. Which of the following manifestations should the nurse identify as an indication of magnesium sulfate toxicity? (Select all that apply.)

   A. Respirations less than 12/min

   B. Urinary output less than 30 mL/hr

   C. Hyperreflexic deep tendon reflexes

   D. Decreased level of consciousness

   E. Flushing and sweating

4. A nursing is assisting in the care of a client who is receiving magnesium sulfate via continuous IV infusion. Which of the following medications should the nurse anticipate administering if magnesium sulfate toxicity is suspected?

   A. Nifedipine

   B. Pyridoxine

   C. Ferrous sulfate

   D. Calcium gluconate

5. A nurse is reviewing a new prescription for ferrous sulfate with a client who is at 12 weeks of gestation. Which of the following statements by the client indicates understanding of the teaching?

   A. "I will take this pill with my breakfast."

   B. "I will take this medication with a glass of milk."

   C. "I plan to drink more orange juice while taking this pill."

   D. "I plan to add more calcium-rich foods to my diet while taking this medication."

PRACTICE Active Learning Scenario

A nurse is reinforcing preprocedure teaching with a client who is at 20 weeks of gestation about prophylactic cervical cerclage. What information should the nurse include? Use the ATI Active Learning Template: Therapeutic Procedure to complete this item.

DESCRIPTION OF PROCEDURE

POTENTIAL COMPLICATIONS: Identify two.

CLIENT EDUCATION: Describe at least four instructions to give the client.

Application Exercises Key

1. A. **CORRECT:** Obesity is a risk factor for hyperemesis gravidarum.

   B. **CORRECT:** Multifetal pregnancy is a risk factor for hyperemesis gravidarum.

   C. Maternal age less than 30 is a risk factor for hyperemesis gravidarum.

   D. Migraine headache is not a risk factor for hyperemesis gravidarum.

   E. Oligohydramnios is not a risk factor for hyperemesis gravidarum.

   (N) *NCLEX® Connection: Health Promotion and Maintenance, Health Promotion/Disease Prevention*

2. A. Altered hematocrit is a manifestation of hyperemesis gravidarum due to the hemoconcentration that occurs with dehydration.

   B. **CORRECT:** The presence of ketones in the urine is associated with the breakdown of proteins and fats that occurs in a client who has hyperemesis gravidarum.

   C. Liver enzymes are elevated in a client who has hyperemesis gravidarum. This result is within the expected reference range.

   D. Decreased serum glucose is anticipated in a client who has hyperemesis gravidarum. This result is within the expected reference range.

   (N) *NCLEX® Connection: Reduction of Risk Potential, Laboratory Values*

3. A. **CORRECT:** A respiratory rate less than 12/min is a manifestation of magnesium sulfate toxicity.

   B. **CORRECT:** Urinary output less than 30 mL/hr is a manifestation of magnesium sulfate toxicity.

   C. The absence of patellar deep tendon reflexes is a manifestation of magnesium sulfate toxicity.

   D. **CORRECT:** Decreased level of consciousness is a manifestation of magnesium sulfate toxicity.

   E. Flushing and sweating are adverse effects of magnesium sulfate but are not manifestations of toxicity.

   (N) *NCLEX® Connection: Pharmacological Therapies, Adverse Effects/ Contraindications/Side Effects/Interactions*

4. A. Nifedipine is an antihypertensive medication that can be administered to clients who have gestational hypertension.

   B. Pyridoxine (vitamin B$_6$) is a vitamin supplement prescribed for clients who have hyperemesis gravidarum.

   C. Ferrous sulfate is a medication used in the treatment of iron deficiency anemia.

   D. **CORRECT:** Calcium gluconate is the antidote for magnesium sulfate.

   (N) *NCLEX® Connection: Pharmacological Therapies, Medication Administration*

5. A. Ferrous sulfate should be taken on an empty stomach.

   B. Milk decreases the absorption of ferrous sulfate.

   C. **CORRECT:** A diet with increased vitamin C improves the absorption of ferrous sulfate.

   D. Although a diet of calcium-rich foods is appropriate for the client during pregnancy, it does not improve the effectiveness of ferrous sulfate.

   (N) *NCLEX® Connection: Pharmacological Therapies, Expected Actions/Outcomes*

PRACTICE Answer

Using the ATI Active Learning Template: Therapeutic Procedure

DESCRIPTION OF PROCEDURE: Surgical reinforcement of the cervix with a suture that is placed around the cervix to strengthen it and prevent premature cervical dilation

CLIENT EDUCATION: Reinforce the following.
- Remain on activity restrictions/bed rest as prescribed.
- Increase hydration to promote a relaxed uterus.
- Refrain from sexual intercourse.
- Findings to report to the provider include preterm labor, rupture of membranes, manifestations of infection, strong contractions less than 5 min apart, perineal pressure, and the urge to push.
- Use of home uterine activity monitor.
- Home health facility to follow up.
- Plan for removal of the cerclage at 37 weeks of gestation.

POTENTIAL COMPLICATIONS
- Uterine contractions
- Rupture of membranes
- Infection

(N) *NCLEX® Connection: Reduction of Risk Potential, Potential for Complications of Diagnostic Tests/Treatments/Procedures*

UNIT 1   ANTEPARTUM NURSING CARE
SECTION: COMPLICATIONS OF PREGNANCY

CHAPTER 9   *Early Onset of Labor*

Understanding the importance of identifying the onset of early labor in a client who is pregnant is crucial for maternal and fetal well-being. This chapter includes preterm labor, premature rupture of membranes, and preterm premature rupture of membranes.

Preterm labor

Preterm labor is uterine contractions and cervical changes that occur between 20 and 37 weeks of gestation.

DATA COLLECTION

RISK FACTORS

- Infections of the urinary tract, vagina, or chorioamnionitis (infection of the amniotic sac)
- Previous preterm birth
- Multifetal pregnancy
- Hydramnios (excessive amniotic fluid)
- Age younger than 17 or older than 35
- Low socioeconomic status
- Smoking
- Substance use
- Intimate partner violence
- History of multiple miscarriages or abortions
- Diabetes mellitus
- Chronic hypertension
- Preeclampsia
- Lack of prenatal care
- Recurrent premature dilation of the cervix
- Placenta previa or abruptio placentae
- Preterm premature rupture of membranes
- Short interval between pregnancies

EXPECTED FINDINGS

- Uterine contractions
- Pressure in the pelvis and menstrual-like cramping
- Persistent low backache
- Gastrointestinal cramping, sometimes with diarrhea
- Urinary frequency
- Vaginal discharge

PHYSICAL FINDINGS

- Increase, change, odor, or blood in vaginal discharge
- Change in cervical dilation
- Regular uterine contractions with a frequency of every 10 min or greater, lasting 1 hr or longer
- Premature rupture of membranes

LABORATORY TESTS

- Fetal fibronectin
- Cervical cultures
- CBC
- Urinalysis

DIAGNOSTIC PROCEDURES

- Obtain swab of vaginal secretions for fetal fibronectin between 24 and 34 weeks of gestation. This protein can be found in vaginal secretions and can be related to inflammation of the placenta that can lead to preterm birth. This test is used to rule out preterm labor.
- Measure endocervical length with an ultrasound to check for a shortened cervix, which is suggested in certain studies to precede preterm labor.
- Obtain cervical cultures to detect if there is a presence of infectious organisms. Culture and sensitivity results guide prescription of proper antibiotics.
- Perform a biophysical profile or a nonstress test to provide information about the fetal well-being.

PATIENT-CENTERED CARE

NURSING CARE

Management of a client who is in preterm labor includes focusing on stopping uterine contractions.

Activity restriction
- Instruct the client on ways to modify the environment to allow for modified bed rest, yet have the ability to fulfill role responsibilities. Strict bed rest can have adverse effects. Q EBP
- Encourage the client to rest in the left lateral position to increase blood flow to the uterus and decrease uterine activity. Q EBP
- Tell the client to avoid sexual intercourse.

Ensuring hydration: Dehydration stimulates the pituitary gland to secrete an antidiuretic hormone and oxytocin. Preventing dehydration prevents the release of oxytocin, which stimulates uterine contractions.

Identifying and treating an infection
- Have the client report any vaginal discharge, noting amount, color, consistency, and odor.
- Monitor vital signs and temperature.

Chorioamnionitis should be suspected with the occurrence of elevated temperature and tachycardia.

Monitor FHR and contraction pattern.

Fetal tachycardia, which is a prolonged increase in the FHR greater than 160/min can indicate infection, is frequently associated with preterm labor.

MEDICATIONS

Nifedipine

CLASSIFICATION AND THERAPEUTIC INTENT: A calcium channel blocker that is used to suppress contractions by inhibiting calcium from entering smooth muscles

NURSING ACTIONS
- Monitor for headache, flushing, dizziness, and nausea. These usually are related to orthostatic hypotension that occurs with administration.
- Do not administer concurrently with magnesium sulfate, or concurrent or immediately following a beta₂ adrenergic agonist. Qs

CLIENT EDUCATION Qs
- Slowly change positions from supine to upright, and sit until dizziness disappears.
- Maintain adequate hydration to counter hypotension.

Magnesium sulfate

CLASSIFICATION AND THERAPEUTIC INTENT: A commonly used tocolytic that suppresses uterine contractions by relaxing the smooth muscle of the uterus

NURSING ACTIONS
- Contraindications for tocolysis include active vaginal bleeding, dilation of the cervix greater than 6 cm, chorioamnionitis, greater than 34 weeks of gestation, and acute fetal distress.
- Monitor the client closely. Discontinue tocolytic therapy immediately if the client exhibits manifestations of pulmonary edema (chest pain, shortness of breath, respiratory distress, audible wheezing and crackles, productive cough containing blood-tinged sputum).
- Monitor for adverse effects.
- Monitor for magnesium sulfate toxicity, and discontinue for any of the following adverse effects: loss of deep tendon reflexes, urinary output less than 30 mL/hr, respiratory depression (less than 12/min), pulmonary edema, and chest pain. Qs
- Administer calcium gluconate or calcium chloride as an antidote for magnesium sulfate toxicity.

CLIENT EDUCATION: Notify the nurse of blurred vision, headache, nausea, vomiting, or difficulty breathing.

Indomethacin

CLASSIFICATION AND THERAPEUTIC INTENT: A nonsteroidal anti-inflammatory drug (NSAID) that suppresses preterm labor by blocking the production of prostaglandins. This inhibition of prostaglandins suppresses uterine contractions.

NURSING ACTIONS
- Monitor the client closely. Discontinue tocolytic therapy immediately if the client exhibits manifestations of pulmonary edema (chest pain, shortness of breath, respiratory distress, audible wheezing and crackles, productive cough containing blood-tinged sputum).
- Indomethacin treatment should not exceed 48 hr.
- Indomethacin should only be used for less than 32 weeks of gestation.

- Monitor for postpartum hemorrhage related to reduced platelet aggregation.
- Administer indomethacin with food or rectally to decrease gastrointestinal distress.
- Monitor the neonate at birth.

Betamethasone

CLASSIFICATION AND THERAPEUTIC INTENT: A glucocorticoid that is administered IM in two injections 24 hr apart and requires 24 hr to be effective. The therapeutic action is to enhance fetal lung maturity and surfactant production in fetuses between 24 to 34 weeks gestation.

NURSING ACTIONS
- Administer the medication deep into the gluteal muscle 24 and 48 hr prior to birth of a preterm neonate.
- Monitor the client and neonate for pulmonary edema by monitoring lung sounds.
- Monitor for maternal and neonate hyperglycemia.
- Monitor the neonate for heart rate changes.

Premature rupture of membranes and preterm premature rupture of membranes

Premature rupture of membranes (PROM) is the spontaneous rupture of the amniotic membranes 1 hr or more prior to the onset of true labor. For most clients, PROM signifies the onset of true labor if gestational duration is at term.

Preterm premature rupture of membranes (PPROM) is the premature spontaneous rupture of membranes after 20 weeks of gestation and prior to 37 weeks of gestation.

DATA COLLECTION

RISK FACTORS

- Infection is a major risk of PROM and PPROM for the client and the fetus. Once the amniotic membranes have ruptured, micro-organisms can ascend from the vagina into the amniotic sac. Infection often precedes PPROM.
- Chorioamnionitis is an infection of the amniotic membranes.
  - There is an increased risk of infection if there is a lag period over the 24-hr period from when the membranes rupture to delivery.
  - History of prior preterm birth
  - Second and third trimester bleeding
  - Uterine overdistention

EXPECTED FINDINGS

Client reports a gush or leakage of clear fluid from the vagina.

PHYSICAL FINDINGS
- Temperature elevation
- Increased maternal heart rate or FHR
- Foul-smelling fluid or vaginal discharge
- Abdominal tenderness

LABORATORY TESTS

- A positive nitrazine paper test (blue, pH 6.5 to 7.5) or positive ferning test is conducted on amniotic fluid to verify rupture of membranes.
- CBC

PATIENT-CENTERED CARE

NURSING CARE

- Prepare for birth if indicated.
- Nursing management depends on gestational duration, if there is evidence of infection, or an indication of fetal or maternal compromise.
- Obtain vaginal/rectal cultures for streptococcus beta-hemolytic.
- Obtain vaginal cultures for chlamydia and *Neisseria gonorrhoeae*.
- Avoid vaginal exams.
- Provide reassurance to reduce anxiety.
- Check vital signs every 2 hr. Notify the provider of a temperature greater than 38° C (100.4° F).
- Monitor FHR and uterine contractions.
- Advise the client to adhere to bed rest with bathroom privileges.
- Encourage hydration.
- Instruct the client to perform daily fetal kick counts and to notify the nurse of uterine contractions.

MEDICATIONS

Ampicillin

CLASSIFICATION AND THERAPEUTIC INTENT: An antibiotic used to treat infection. It is commonly used to treat chorioamnionitis.

NURSING ACTIONS: Obtain vaginal, urine, and blood cultures prior to administration of antibiotic.

Betamethasone

CLASSIFICATION AND THERAPEUTIC INTENT: A glucocorticoid administered IM in two injections, 24 hr apart, and requires 24 hr to be effective. It enhances fetal lung maturity and surfactant production.

NURSING ACTIONS
- Administer the medication deep into the gluteal muscle 24 and 48 hr prior to birth of a preterm neonate.
- Monitor the client and neonate for pulmonary edema by monitoring lung sounds.
- Monitor for maternal and neonate hyperglycemia.
- Monitor the neonate for heart rate changes.

CLIENT EDUCATION

- Expect to be discharged home if dilation is less than 3 cm, no evidence of infection, no contractions, and no malpresentation.
- Adhere to limited activity with bathroom privileges.
- Encourage hydration.
- Conduct a self-assessment for uterine contractions.
- Record daily kick counts for fetal movement.
- Monitor for foul-smelling vaginal discharge.
- Refrain from inserting anything into the vagina.
- Abstain from intercourse.
- Avoid tub baths.
- Wipe perineal area from front to back after voiding and fecal elimination.
- Take temperature every 4 hr when awake and report a temperature that is greater than 38° C (100° F).

Application Exercises

1. A nurse is reviewing the medical record of a client who reports indications of preterm labor. Which of the following client findings are risk factors for this condition? (Select all that apply).

   A. Urinary tract infection
   B. Multifetal pregnancy
   C. Oligohydramnios
   D. Diabetes mellitus
   E. Uterine abnormalities

2. A nurse is assisting with the care of a client who is in preterm labor at 32 weeks of gestation. Which of the following medications should the nurse expect the provider to prescribe to hasten fetal lung maturity?

   A. Calcium gluconate
   B. Indomethacin
   C. Nifedipine
   D. Betamethasone

3. A nurse is assisting with the care of a client who is receiving nifedipine for prevention of preterm labor. The nurse should monitor the client for which of the following manifestations?

   A. Blood-tinged sputum
   B. Dizziness
   C. Pallor
   D. Somnolence

4. A nurse is assisting with the care of a client who has a prescription for magnesium sulfate. The nurse should recognize that which of the following are contraindications for use of this medication? (Select all that apply.)

   A. Fetal distress
   B. Preterm labor
   C. Vaginal bleeding
   D. Cervical dilation greater than 6 cm
   E. Severe gestational hypertension

5. A nurse is reinforcing discharge teaching with a client who experienced premature rupture of membranes at 26 weeks of gestation. Which of the following information should the nurse include in the instructions?

   A. Use a condom with sexual intercourse.
   B. Avoid bubble bath solution when taking a tub bath.
   C. Wipe from the back to front when performing perineal hygiene.
   D. Keep a daily record of fetal kick counts.

PRACTICE Active Learning Scenario

A nurse in a prenatal clinic is reviewing preterm labor with a newly hired nurse. Which of the following information should the nurse include in the discussion? Use the ATI Active Learning Template: System Disorder to complete this item.

ALTERATION IN HEALTH (DIAGNOSIS)

EXPECTED FINDINGS: Describe at least six manifestations.

DIAGNOSTIC PROCEDURES: Describe at least three.

Application Exercises Key

1. A. **CORRECT:** A urinary tract infection is a risk factor of preterm labor.

   B. **CORRECT:** Multifetal pregnancy is a risk factor of preterm labor.

   C. Hydramnios (excessive amniotic fluid) is a risk factor for preterm labor.

   D. **CORRECT:** Diabetes mellitus is a risk factor of preterm labor.

   E. **CORRECT:** Uterine abnormalities are a risk factor of preterm labor.

   Ⓝ *NCLEX® Connection: Health Promotion and Maintenance, Health Promotion/Disease Prevention*

2. A. Calcium gluconate is administered as an antidote for magnesium sulfate toxicity.

   B. Indomethacin is an NSAID used to suppress preterm labor by blocking prostaglandin production.

   C. Nifedipine is a calcium channel blocker used to suppress uterine contractions.

   D. **CORRECT:** Betamethasone is a glucocorticoid given to clients in preterm labor to hasten surfactant production.

   Ⓝ *NCLEX® Connection: Pharmacological Therapies, Medication Administration*

3. A. Blood-tinged sputum production is an adverse effect associated with indomethacin.

   B. **CORRECT:** Dizziness and lightheadedness are associated with orthostatic hypotension, which occurs when taking nifedipine.

   C. Facial flushing and heat sensation are adverse effects associated with nifedipine.

   D. Nervousness, jitteriness, and sleep disturbances are adverse effects associated with nifedipine.

   Ⓝ *NCLEX® Connection: Pharmacological Therapies, Adverse Effects/ Contraindications/Side Effects/Interactions*

4. A. **CORRECT:** Acute fetal distress is a contraindication for use of magnesium sulfate therapy.

   B. Preterm labor is an indication for use of magnesium sulfate.

   C. **CORRECT:** Vaginal bleeding is a contraindication for magnesium sulfate therapy.

   D. **CORRECT:** Cervical dilation greater than 6 cm is a contraindication for magnesium sulfate therapy.

   E. Severe gestational hypertension is an indication for the use of magnesium sulfate.

   Ⓝ *NCLEX® Connection: Pharmacological Therapies, Adverse Effects/ Contraindications/Side Effects/Interactions*

5. A. The client who has ruptured membranes should not insert anything into the vagina.

   B. The nurse should instruct the client to avoid tub baths and take showers.

   C. The nurse should instruct the client to wipe from front to back when performing perineal hygiene.

   D. **CORRECT:** The client should record daily fetal kick counts.

   Ⓝ *NCLEX® Connection: Physiological Adaptation, Alterations in Body Systems*

PRACTICE Answer

Using the ATI Active Learning Template: System Disorder

ALTERATION IN HEALTH (DIAGNOSIS): Uterine contractions and cervical changes that occur between 20 and 37 weeks of gestation

EXPECTED FINDINGS
- Persistent low backache
- Pressure in the pelvis and cramping
- Gastrointestinal cramping, sometimes with diarrhea
- Urinary frequency
- Vaginal discharge
- Increase, change, or blood in vaginal discharge
- Change in cervical dilation
- Regular uterine contractions with a frequency of every 10 min or greater, lasting 1 hr or longer
- Premature rupture of membranes

DIAGNOSTIC PROCEDURES
- Test for fetal fibronectin
- Ultrasound to measure endocervical length
- Cervical culture to detect presence of infectious organisms
- Biophysical profile
- Nonstress test
- Home uterine activity monitoring for uterine contractions

Ⓝ *NCLEX® Connection: Reduction of Risk Potential, Potential for Alterations in Body Systems*

NCLEX® Connections

When reviewing the following chapters, keep in mind the relevant topics and tasks of the NCLEX outline, in particular:

Health Promotion and Maintenance

ANTE/INTRA/POSTPARTUM AND NEWBORN CARE
Assist with monitoring a client in labor.

Assist with fetal heart monitoring for the antepartum client.

DATA COLLECTION TECHNIQUES: Prepare client for physical examination (reinforce explanation of procedure, provide privacy and comfort).

Basic Care and Comfort

NONPHARMACOLOGICAL COMFORT INTERVENTIONS: Provide nonpharmacological measures for pain relief (imagery, massage or repositioning).

Pharmacological Therapies

ADVERSE EFFECTS/CONTRAINDICATIONS/ SIDE EFFECTS/INTERACTIONS: Monitor and document client side effects to medications.

PHARMACOLOGICAL PAIN MANAGEMENT: Maintain pain control devices (epidural, patient control analgesia, peripheral nerve catheter).

Physiological Adaptation

ALTERATIONS IN BODY SYSTEMS
Provide care for a client experiencing complications of pregnancy/ labor and/or delivery (eclampsia, precipitous labor, hemorrhage).

Notify the primary health care provider of a change in the client's status.

MEDICAL EMERGENCIES: Respond/intervene to a client's life-threatening situation (cardiopulmonary resuscitation).

UNIT 2   INTRAPARTUM NURSING CARE

CHAPTER 10 *Nursing Care of the Client in Labor*

An intrapartum nurse should care for three clients during each labor and delivery: the fetus, mother, and family unit. **(10.1)**

DATA COLLECTION

An intrapartum nurse should collect data on maternal and fetal well-being during labor, the progress of labor, and psychosocial and cultural factors that affect labor. Q**PCC**

PHYSIOLOGIC CHANGES PRECEDING LABOR (PREMONITORY SIGNS)

Backache: Constant low, dull backache caused by pelvic muscle relaxation

Weight loss: 0.5 to 1.5 kg (1 to 3.5 lb)

Lightening: Fetal head descends into true pelvis about 14 days before labor
- Feeling that the fetus has "dropped"
- Easier breathing, but more pressure on bladder, resulting in urinary frequency
- More pronounced in clients who are primigravida

Contractions: Begin with irregular uterine contractions (Braxton Hicks) that eventually progress in strength and regularity

Increased vaginal discharge or bloody show: Expulsion of the cervical mucus plug can occur. Brownish or blood-tinged mucus plug resulting from the onset of cervical dilation and effacement.

Energy burst: Sometimes called "nesting" response

Gastrointestinal changes: Less common; include nausea, vomiting, and indigestion

Cervical ripening: Cervix becomes soft and partially effaced, and can begin to dilate

Rupture of membranes: Spontaneous rupture of membranes can initiate labor or can occur anytime during labor, most commonly during the transition phase.
- Labor usually occurs within 24 hr of the rupture of membranes.
- Prolonged rupture of membranes greater than 24 hr before delivery of fetus can lead to an infection.
- Immediately following the rupture of membranes, a nurse should check the FHR for abrupt decelerations, which are indicative of fetal distress to rule out umbilical cord prolapse. Q**s**

Evaluation of amniotic fluid: Completed once the membranes rupture
- Should be watery, clear, and pale- to straw-yellow in color.
- Odor should not be foul.
- Volume is 500 to 1,200 mL.
- Use nitrazine paper to confirm presence of amniotic fluid.
  ○ **Amniotic fluid is alkaline:** Nitrazine paper is deep blue, indicating pH of 6.5 to 7.5.
  ○ **Urine is slightly acidic:** Nitrazine paper remains yellow.

FIVE P's

Five factors affect and define the labor and birth process.
- **Passenger** (fetus and placenta)
- **Passageway** (birth canal)
- **Powers** (contractions)
- **Position** (of the client)
- **Psychological** response

Passenger

Consists of the fetus and the placenta. The size of the fetal head, fetal presentation, fetal lie, fetal attitude, and fetal position affect the ability of the fetus to navigate the birth canal. The placenta can be considered a passenger because it also must pass through the canal.

Presentation: The part of the fetus that is entering the pelvic inlet first and leads through the birth canal during labor. It can be the back of the head (occiput), chin (mentum), shoulder (scapula), or breech (sacrum or feet).

Lie: The relationship of the maternal longitudinal axis (spine) to the fetal longitudinal axis (spine)
- **Transverse:** Fetal long axis is horizontal, forms a right angle to maternal axis, and will not accommodate vaginal birth. The shoulder is the presenting part and can require delivery by cesarean birth if the fetus does not rotate spontaneously.
- **Parallel or longitudinal:** Fetal long axis is parallel to maternal long axis, either cephalic or breech presentation. Breech presentation can require a cesarean birth.

Attitude: Relationship of fetal body parts to one another
- **Fetal flexion:** Chin flexed to chest, extremities flexed into torso
- **Fetal extension:** Chin extended away from chest, extremities extended

Fetopelvic or fetal position: The relationship of the presenting part of the fetus (sacrum, mentum, occiput), preferably the occiput, in reference to its directional position as it relates to one of the four maternal pelvic quadrants. It is labeled with three letters.
- **Right (R) or left (L):** The first letter references the side of the maternal pelvis.
- **Occiput (O), sacrum (S), mentum (M), or scapula (Sc):** The second letter references the presenting part of the fetus.
- **Anterior (A), posterior (P), or transverse (T):** The third letter references the part of the maternal pelvis.

Station: Measurement of fetal descent in centimeters
- Station 0 at the level of an imaginary line at the level of the ischial spines
- Minus stations superior to the ischial spines
- Plus stations inferior to the ischial spines

Passageway

The birth canal is composed of the bony pelvis, cervix, pelvic floor, vagina, and introitus (vaginal opening). The size and shape of the bony pelvis must be adequate to allow the fetus to pass through it. The cervix must dilate and efface in response to contractions and fetal descent.

Powers

Uterine contractions cause effacement (shortening and thinning of the cervix) during the first stage of labor and dilation of the cervix (enlargement or widening of the cervical opening and canal) that occurs once labor has begun and the fetus is descending. Involuntary urge to push and voluntary bearing down in the second stage of labor helps in the expulsion of the fetus.

Position

The client should engage in frequent position changes during labor to increase comfort, relieve fatigue, and promote circulation. Position during the second stage is determined by maternal preference, provider preference, and condition of the mother and fetus.

Gravity can aid in fetal descent in upright, sitting, kneeling, and squatting positions.

Psychological response

Maternal stress, tension, and anxiety can produce physiological changes that impair the progress of labor.

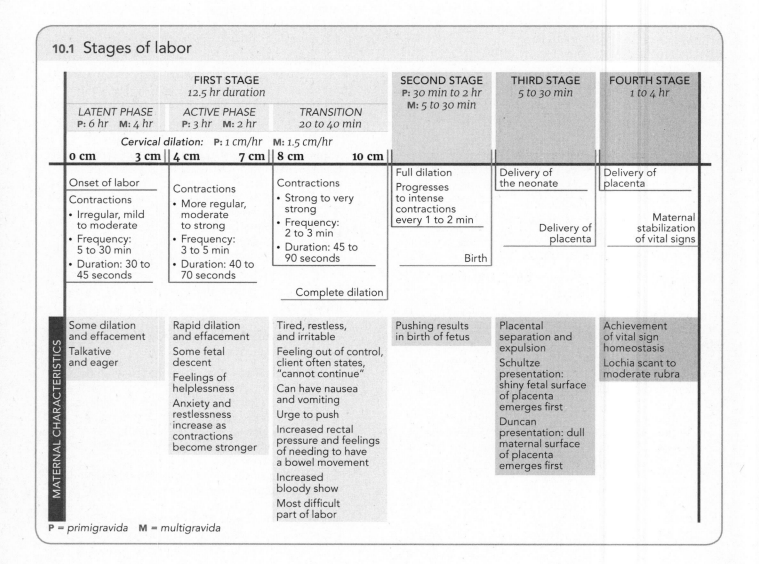

10.1 Stages of labor

	FIRST STAGE *12.5 hr duration*			SECOND STAGE P: 30 min to 2 hr M: 5 to 30 min	THIRD STAGE 5 to 30 min	FOURTH STAGE 1 to 4 hr
	LATENT PHASE P: 6 hr M: 4 hr	*ACTIVE PHASE* P: 3 hr M: 2 hr	*TRANSITION* 20 to 40 min			
	Cervical dilation: P: 1 cm/hr M: 1.5 cm/hr					
	0 cm 3 cm	**4 cm 7 cm**	**8 cm 10 cm**			
	Onset of labor Contractions • Irregular, mild to moderate • Frequency: 5 to 30 min • Duration: 30 to 45 seconds	Contractions • More regular, moderate to strong • Frequency: 3 to 5 min • Duration: 40 to 70 seconds	Contractions • Strong to very strong • Frequency: 2 to 3 min • Duration: 45 to 90 seconds Complete dilation	Full dilation Progresses to intense contractions every 1 to 2 min Birth	Delivery of the neonate Delivery of placenta	Delivery of placenta Maternal stabilization of vital signs
MATERNAL CHARACTERISTICS	Some dilation and effacement Talkative and eager	Rapid dilation and effacement Some fetal descent Feelings of helplessness Anxiety and restlessness increase as contractions become stronger	Tired, restless, and irritable Feeling out of control, client often states, "cannot continue" Can have nausea and vomiting Urge to push Increased rectal pressure and feelings of needing to have a bowel movement Increased bloody show Most difficult part of labor	Pushing results in birth of fetus	Placental separation and expulsion Schultze presentation: shiny fetal surface of placenta emerges first Duncan presentation: dull maternal surface of placenta emerges first	Achievement of vital sign homeostasis Lochia scant to moderate rubra

P = primigravida   **M** = multigravida

PATIENT-CENTERED CARE

PREPROCEDURE

NURSING CARE

- **External electronic monitoring (tocotransducer):** Separate transducer applied to the maternal abdomen over the fundus that measures uterine activity
  - Displays uterine contraction patterns
  - Easily applied by the nurse but must be repositioned with maternal movement to ensure proper placement
- **External fetal monitoring (EFM):** Transducer applied to the abdomen of the client to monitor FHR patterns during labor and birth

LABORATORY ANALYSIS

- **Group B streptococcus:** Culture is obtained if results are not available from screening at 35 to 37 weeks. If positive, IV prophylactic antibiotic is prescribed. (Exceptions are planned cesarean birth and membranes intact.) Qs
- **Urinalysis:** Clean-catch urine sample obtained to ascertain maternal:
  - Hydration status via specific gravity
  - Nutritional status via ketones
  - Proteinuria, which can be indicative of gestational hypertension or pre-eclampsia
  - Glucosuria, which can be indicative of gestational diabetes
  - Urinary tract infection (UTI) via bacterial count (UTIs are common in a diabetic pregnancy)
- **Blood tests**
  - CBC level
  - ABO typing and Rh-factor if not previously done

NURSING ACTIONS: Provide the client and partner with ongoing education regarding the labor and delivery process and procedures.

INTRAPROCEDURE

NURSING CARE

- **Check maternal vital signs** per agency protocol. Check maternal temperature every 1 to 2 hr if membranes are ruptured.
- **Monitor FHR** to determine fetal well-being. This can be performed by use of EFM or spiral electrode that is applied to the fetal scalp by a registered nurse trained in the procedure or the provider. Prior to electrode placement, cervical dilation and rupture of membranes must occur.
- **Monitor uterine labor contraction characteristics** by palpation (placing a hand over the fundus to evaluate contraction frequency, duration, and intensity) or use of external or internal monitoring. **(10.2)**
  - **Frequency:** Established from the beginning of one contraction to the beginning of the next
  - **Duration:** Time between the beginning of a contraction to the end of that same contraction
  - **Intensity:** Strength of the contraction at its peak, described as mild (slightly tense, like pressing finger to tip of nose), moderate (firm, like pressing finger to chin), or strong (rigid, like pressing finger to forehead)
  - **Resting tone of uterine contractions:** Tone of the uterine muscle in between contractions. A prolonged contraction duration (greater than 90 seconds) or too frequent contractions (more than five in a 10-min period) without sufficient time for uterine relaxation (less than 30 seconds) in between can reduce blood flow to the placenta. This can result in fetal hypoxia and changes FHR. Qs

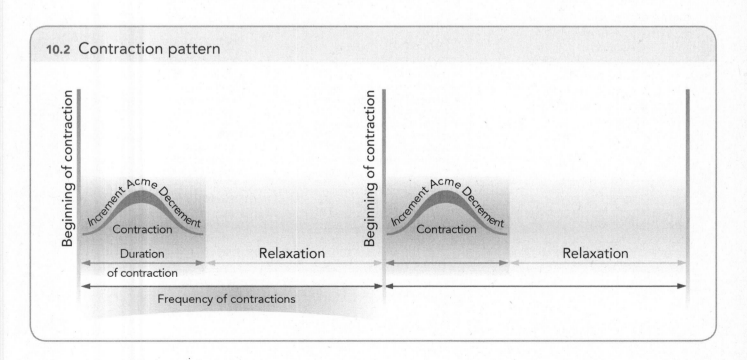

10.2 Contraction pattern

Beginning of contraction — Increment Acme Decrement / Contraction — Duration of contraction — Relaxation — Frequency of contractions

Beginning of contraction — Increment Acme Decrement / Contraction — Relaxation

- **Vaginal examination:** Performed digitally by the provider or qualified nurse to check for the following.
  - Cervical dilation (stretching of cervical os adequate to allow fetal passage) and effacement (cervical thinning and shortening) **(10.3)**
  - Descent of the fetus through the birth canal as measured by fetal station in centimeters
  - Fetal position, presenting part, and lie
  - Membranes that are intact or ruptured
- **Mechanism of labor in vertex presentation:** The adaptations the fetus makes as it progresses through the birth canal during the birthing process
  - **Engagement:** Occurs when the presenting part—usually biparietal (largest) diameter—of the fetal head passes the pelvic inlet at the level of the ischial spines, referred to as station 0.
  - **Descent:** The progress of the presenting part (preferably the occiput) through the pelvis. Measured by station during a vaginal examination as either minus (–) station measured in centimeters if superior to station 0 and not yet engaged, or plus (+) station measured in centimeters if inferior to station 0.
  - **Flexion:** When the fetal head meets resistance of the cervix, pelvic wall, or pelvic floor. The head flexes, bringing the chin close to the chest, presenting a smaller diameter to pass through the pelvis.
  - **Internal rotation:** The fetal occiput ideally rotates to a lateral anterior position as it progresses from the ischial spines to the lower pelvis in a corkscrew motion to pass through the pelvis.
  - **Extension:** The fetal occiput passes under the symphysis pubis, and then the head is deflected anteriorly and is born by extension of the chin away from the fetal chest.
  - **External rotation (restitution):** After the head is born, it rotates to the position it occupied as it entered the pelvic inlet (restitution) in alignment with the fetal body and completes a quarter turn to face transverse as the anterior shoulder passes under the symphysis.
  - **Birth by expulsion:** After birth of the head and shoulders, the trunk of the neonate is born by flexing it toward the symphysis pubis.

POSTPROCEDURE

NURSING DATA COLLECTION DURING THE FOURTH STAGE
- Maternal vital signs
- Fundus
- Lochia
- Perineum
- Urinary output
- Maternal/newborn baby-friendly activities

NURSING INTERVENTIONS DURING THE FOURTH STAGE
- American Academy of Pediatrics and American Congress of Obstetricians and Gynecologists recommend that blood pressure and pulse be checked at least every 15 min for the first 2 hr after birth, and that temperature be monitored every 4 hr for the first 8 hr after birth and then at least every 8 hr.
- Check fundus and lochia every 15 min for the first hour and then according to facility protocol.
- Massage the uterine fundus and/or ensure administration of oxytocics by a qualified nurse to maintain uterine tone to prevent hemorrhage. Qs
- Check the client's perineum, and provide comfort measures.
- Encourage voiding to prevent bladder distention.
- Promote an opportunity for maternal/newborn bonding.
- Offer assistance with breastfeeding, and provide reassurance.

CLIENT EDUCATION: Notify the nurse of increased vaginal bleeding or passage of blood clots.

10.3 Characteristics of true vs. false labor

True labor leads to cervical dilation and effacement.

True labor	*False labor*
CONTRACTIONS	**CONTRACTIONS**
• Can begin irregularly, but become regular in frequency	• Painless, irregular frequency, and intermittent
• Stronger, last longer, and are more frequent	• Decrease in frequency, duration, and intensity with walking or position changes
• Felt in lower back, radiating to abdomen	• Felt in lower back or abdomen above umbilicus
• Walking can increase contraction intensity	• Often stop with sleep or comfort measures such as oral hydration or emptying of the bladder
• Continue despite comfort measures	
CERVIX (determined by vaginal exam)	**CERVIX** (determined by vaginal exam)
• Progressive change in dilation and effacement	• No significant change in dilation or effacement
• Moves to anterior position	• Often remains in posterior position
• Bloody show	• No significant bloody show
FETUS: Presenting part engages in pelvis	**FETUS:** Presenting part is not engaged in pelvis

Pain Management

Pain is a subjective and individual experience. Each client's response to the pain of labor is unique. Safety for the mother and fetus must be the first consideration of the nurse when planning pain management measures. Qs

SOURCES OF PAIN DURING LABOR

First stage

Internal visceral pain that can be felt as back and leg pain

PAIN CAUSES
- Dilation, effacement, and stretching of the cervix
- Distention of the lower segment of the uterus
- Contractions of the uterus with resultant uterine ischemia

Second stage

Pain that is somatic and occurs with fetal descent and expulsion

PAIN CAUSES
- Pressure and distention of the vagina and the perineum, described by as "burning," "splitting," and "tearing"
- Pressure and pulling on the pelvic structures (ligaments, fallopian tubes, ovaries, bladder, peritoneum)
- Lacerations of soft tissues (cervix, vagina, perineum)

Third stage

Pain with the expulsion of the placenta is similar to the pain experienced during the first stage.

PAIN CAUSES
- Uterine contractions
- Pressure and pulling of pelvic structures

Fourth stage

Pain is caused by distention and stretching of the vagina and perineum incurred during the second stage with a splitting, burning, and tearing sensation.

PAIN ASSESSMENT

- Pain level cannot always be evaluated by monitoring the outward expressions of a client. Client pain ment can require persistent questioning and astute observation by the nurse. Cultural beliefs and behaviors of clients during labor and delivery can affect the client's pain management.
- Anxiety and fear are associated with pain. As fear and anxiety increase, muscle tension increases, and thus the experience of pain increases, becoming a cycle of pain. Fear, tension, and pain slow the progression of labor.
- Check beliefs and expectations related to discomfort, pain relief, and birth plans regarding pain relief methods for clients in labor.
- Check level, quality, frequency, duration, intensity, and location of pain through verbal and nonverbal cues. Use an appropriate pain scale allowing the client to indicate the severity of her pain on a scale of 0 to 10, with 10 representing the most severe pain.
- INDICATIONS OF PAIN
  - Behavioral manifestations (crying, moaning, screaming, gesturing, writhing, avoidance or withdrawal, inability to follow instructions)
  - Increasing blood pressure, tachycardia, and hyperventilation
- The nurse is responsible for assisting the client with positioning for comfort during labor and birth, and following pharmacological interventions.
- A nurse should provide client safety after any pharmacological intervention by putting the bed in a low position, maintaining side rails in the up position, placing the call light within the client's reach, and advising the client and her partner to call for assistance if she needs to leave the bed or ambulate. Qs
- Evaluate the client's response to pain relief methods used (verbal report that pain is relieved or being relieved, appears relaxed between contractions). **(10.4)**

10.4 Appropriate pain relief measures during labor

	FIRST STAGE	SECOND STAGE	VAGINAL BIRTH	CESAREAN BIRTH
Opioid agonist analgesics	✓			
Opioid agonist-antagonist analgesics	✓			
Epidural (block) analgesia	✓	✓	✓	
Epidural (block) anesthesia			✓	✓
Combined spinal-epidural (CSE) analgesia	✓		✓	
Nitrous oxide	✓	✓	✓	
Local infiltration anesthesia			✓	✓
Nerve block analgesia and anesthesia		✓		
Pudendal block		✓	✓	
Spinal (block) anesthesia		✓	✓	✓
General anesthesia				✓

NONPHARMACOLOGICAL PAIN MANAGEMENT

Nonpharmacological pain management measures reduce anxiety, fear, and tension, which are major contributing factors to pain in labor.

GATE CONTROL THEORY OF PAIN

- Based on the concept that the sensory nerve pathways that pain sensations use to travel to the brain will allow only a limited number of sensations to travel at any given time. By sending alternate signals through these pathways, the pain signals can be blocked from ascending the neurological pathway and inhibit the brain's perception and sensation of pain.
- Assists in the understanding of how nonpharmacological pain techniques can work to relieve pain.

INTERVENTIONS

Cognitive strategies

- Childbirth education
- Childbirth preparation methods (Lamaze, patterned breathing exercises) promote relaxation and pain management.
- Doulas can assist clients using methods for nonpharmacological pain management.
- Nursing implications include monitoring for findings of hyperventilation (caused by low blood levels of PCO_2 from blowing off too much CO_2), such as lightheadedness and tingling of the fingers. If this occurs, have the client breathe into a paper bag or her cupped hands.
- Hypnosis
- Biofeedback

Sensory stimulation strategies

Based on the gate control theory to promote relaxation and pain relief
- Aromatherapy
- Breathing techniques
- Imagery
- Music
- Use of focal points
- Subdued lighting

Cutaneous stimulation strategies

Based on the gate-control theory to promote relaxation and pain relief
- Therapeutic touch (back rubs, massage)
- Walking
- Rocking
- Effleurage: Light, gentle circular stroking of the client's abdomen with the fingertips in rhythm with breathing during contractions
- Sacral counterpressure: Consistent pressure is applied by the support person using the heel of the hand or fist against the client's sacral area to counteract pain in the lower back
- Application of heat or cold
- Transcutaneous electrical nerve stimulation (TENS) therapy
- Hydrotherapy (whirlpool or shower) increases maternal endorphin levels
- Acupressure
- Frequent maternal position changes to promote relaxation and pain relief
  - Semi-sitting
  - Squatting
  - Kneeling
  - Kneeling and rocking back and forth
  - Supine position only with the placement of a wedge under one of the client's hips to tilt the uterus and avoid supine hypotension syndrome

CLIENT EDUCATION: Use techniques to promote pain management (patterned breathing, progressive relaxation exercises).

PHARMACOLOGICAL PAIN MANAGEMENT

Includes analgesia and local/regional analgesics. To avoid slowing the progress of labor, prior to administering analgesic medications, the nurse should verify that labor is well established following a vaginal exam by a qualified nurse and evaluation of uterine contraction pattern. Q_{EBP}

Alleviates pain sensations or raises the threshold for pain perception

ANALGESIA

Pharmacological pain interventions

- When given early in the labor process, they can slow or stop labor.
- Monitor maternal vital signs, uterine contraction pattern, and continuous FHR monitoring. Check maternal vital signs and fetal heart rate and pattern. Document before and after administration of pain medications.
- Sedatives (secobarbital, pentobarbital, phenobarbital) are not used during birth. Neonate respiratory depression can occur secondary to the medication crossing the placenta and affecting the fetus. These medications should not be administered if birth is anticipated within 12 to 24 hr.

Opioid analgesics

Opioid analgesics (meperidine hydrochloride, fentanyl, butorphanol, nalbuphine) are usually given during the early part of active labor.

- These medications cross the placental barrier. If given to the mother too close to the time of delivery, opioid analgesics can cause respiratory depression in the neonate.
- Prior to administering analgesic medication, verify that labor is well established by a qualified nurse.

Naloxone, an opioid antagonist, should be readily available for reversal of opioid-induced respiratory depression in the client or newborn. Qs

PHARMACOLOGICAL ANESTHESIA

- Pharmacological anesthesia eliminates pain perceptions by interrupting the nerve impulses to the brain.
- Anesthesia used in childbirth includes regional blocks and general anesthesia.

Regional blocks

Regional blocks are most commonly used and consist of pudendal, epidural, spinal, and paracervical nerve block.

Pudendal block

Consists of a local anesthetic (lidocaine, bupivacaine) administered transvaginally into the space in front of the pudendal nerve. This type of block has no maternal or fetal systemic effects, but it does provide local anesthesia to the perineum, vulva, and rectal areas during delivery, episiotomy, and episiotomy repair. It is administered during the late second stage of labor 10 to 20 min before delivery, providing analgesia prior to spontaneous expulsion of the fetus or forceps-assisted or vacuum-assisted birth. It is suitable during the second and third stages of labor and for repair of episiotomy and lacerations.

Epidural block

Consists of a local anesthetic, bupivacaine, along with an analgesic, morphine, or fentanyl, injected into the epidural space at the level of the fourth or fifth lumbar vertebrae. This eliminates all sensation from the level of the umbilicus to the thighs, relieving the discomfort of uterine contractions, fetal descent, and pressure and stretching of the perineum. It is administered when the client is in active labor and dilated to at least 4 cm. Continuous infusion or intermittent injections can be administered through an indwelling epidural catheter. Patient-controlled epidural analgesia is a technique for labor analgesia and is a favored method of pain management for labor and birth. It is suitable for all stages of labor, most types of birth, and repair of episiotomy and lacerations.

Spinal anesthesia (block)

Consists of a local anesthetic that is injected into the subarachnoid space into the spinal fluid at the third, fourth, or fifth lumbar interspace. The spinal block eliminates all sensations from the level of the nipples to the feet. It is commonly used for cesarean births. A low spinal block can be used for a vaginal birth, but it is not used for labor. A spinal block is administered in the late second stage or before cesarean birth.

- ADVERSE EFFECTS
  - Maternal hypotension
  - Fetal bradycardia
  - Inability to feel the urge to void
  - Loss of the bearing down reflex
- NURSING ACTIONS
  - Administer a bolus of IV fluids to help offset maternal hypotension. QEBP
  - Help position and steady the client into a sitting or side-lying modified Sims' position with her back curved to widen the intervertebral space for insertion of the epidural catheter.
  - Encourage the client to remain in the side-lying position after insertion of the epidural catheter to avoid supine hypotension syndrome with compression of the vena cava.
  - Coach the client in pushing efforts, and request an evaluation of epidural pain management by anesthesia personnel if pushing efforts are ineffective.
  - Monitor maternal blood pressure and pulse. Observe for hypotension, respiratory depression, and decreased oxygen saturation.
  - Monitor FHR patterns continuously.
  - Maintain the IV line. Have oxygen and suction available.
  - Provide for client safety, such as by raising the side rails of the bed. Do not allow the client to ambulate.
  - Check the bladder for distention at frequent intervals. Catheterize if necessary to prevent discomfort and interference with uterine contractions.
  - Monitor for the return of sensation and motor control in the client's legs after delivery but prior to standing. Assist the client with standing and walking for the first time after a delivery that included spinal or epidural anesthesia.
  - Potential headache from leakage of cerebrospinal fluid at the puncture site. Encourage interventions to relieve a postpartum headache resulting from a cerebrospinal fluid leak (placing the client in a supine position; promoting bed rest in a dark room; administering oral analgesics, caffeine, fluids). An autologous blood patch is the most beneficial and reliable relief measure for cerebrospinal fluid leaks.

Therapeutic Procedures to Assist with Labor and Delivery

Induction of labor

Induction of labor is the deliberate initiation of uterine contractions to stimulate labor before spontaneous onset to bring about the birth by chemical or mechanical means.

METHODS
- Mechanical or chemical approaches
- Administration of IV oxytocin
- Nipple stimulation to trigger the release of endogenous oxytocin

INDICATIONS

- Any condition in which augmentation or induction of labor is indicated.
- Elective induction for nonmedical indications must meet the criteria of at least 39 weeks of gestation and a Bishop score of greater than 8 for a multiparous client and greater than 10 for a nulliparous.
- Elective inductions that do not meet recommended criteria can result in increased risk for infection, premature delivery, longer labor, and need for cesarean birth.

CLIENT PRESENTATION
- Postterm pregnancy (greater than 42 weeks of gestation)
- Dystocia (prolonged, difficult labor) due to inadequate uterine contractions.
- Prolonged rupture of membranes predisposes the client and fetus to risk of infection.
- Maternal complications
  - Rh-isoimmunization
  - Diabetes mellitus
  - Pulmonary disease
  - Gestational hypertension
- Fetal demise
- Chorioamnionitis

CONSIDERATIONS

Cervical ripening

The client can undergo cervical ripening prior to induction of labor using prostaglandin E_1 or E_2.
- Cervical ripening by various methods increases cervical readiness for labor through promotion of cervical softening, dilation, and effacement.
- Cervical ripening can eliminate the need for oxytocin administration to induce labor, lower the dosage of oxytocin needed, and promote a more successful induction
- Monitor FHR and uterine activity after administration of cervical-ripening agents.
- Notify the provider if uterine hyperstimulation or fetal distress is noted.

Induction of labor

Oxytocin is used to initiate induction.
- When oxytocin is administered, data collection includes maternal blood pressure, pulse, and respirations every 30 to 60 min and with every change in dose.
- Monitor FHR and contraction pattern every 15 min and with every change in dose.
- Evaluate fluid intake and urinary output.
- Oxytocin is discontinued if uterine hyperstimulation occurs.

Manifestations of uterine hyperstimulation Qs
- Contraction frequency more often than every 2 min
- Contraction duration longer than 90 seconds
- Contraction intensity that results in pressures greater than 90 mm Hg as shown by IUPC
- Uterine resting tone greater than 20 mm Hg between contractions
- No relaxation of uterus between contractions

COMPLICATIONS

Nonreassuring FHR

- Abnormal baseline less than 110 or greater than 160/min
- Loss of variability
- Late or prolonged decelerations

NURSING ACTIONS
- Notify the provider.
- Position the client in a side-lying position to increase uteroplacental perfusion.
- Keep the IV line open and increase the rate of IV fluid administration to 200 mL/hr unless contraindicated.
- Administer O_2 by a face mask at 8 to 10 L/min.
- Administer the tocolytic terbutaline 0.25 mg subcutaneously to diminish uterine activity.
- Monitor FHR and patterns in conjunction with uterine activity.
- Document responses to interventions.
- If unable to restore reassuring FHR, prepare for an emergency cesarean birth.

Augmentation of labor

Augmentation of labor is the stimulation of hypotonic contractions once labor has spontaneously begun, but progress is inadequate.

Some providers favor active management of labor to establish effective labor with the aggressive use of oxytocin or rupture of membranes.

RISK FACTORS REQUIRING AUGMENTATION OF LABOR: Administration procedures, nursing data collection and interventions, and possible procedure complications are the same for labor induction.

Amniotomy

- An amniotomy is the artificial rupture of the amniotic membranes (AROM) by the provider using a small hook or other sharp instrument.
- Labor typically begins within 12 hr after the membranes rupture and can decrease the duration of labor by up to 2 hr.
- The client is at an increased risk for cord prolapse or infection.
- An amniotomy is indicated when labor progression is too slow and augmentation or induction of labor is indicated.

CONSIDERATIONS

ONGOING CARE

- The presenting part of the fetus must be engaged prior to an amniotomy to prevent cord prolapse.
- Monitor FHR prior to and immediately following AROM to monitor for cord prolapse as evidenced by variable or late decelerations.
- Evaluate and document characteristics of amniotic fluid including color, odor, and consistency.

NURSING ACTIONS

- Document the time of rupture.
- Obtain temperature every 2 hr.
- Provide comfort measures (frequently change pads, perineal cleansing)

Vacuum-assisted delivery

A vacuum-assisted birth involves the use of a cuplike suction device that is attached to the fetal head. Traction is applied during contractions to assist in the descent and birth of the head, after which the vacuum cup is released and removed preceding delivery of the fetal body.

Follow recommendations by the manufacturer for product use to ensure safety.

CONDITIONS FOR USE

- Vertex presentation
- Absence of cephalopelvic disproportion
- Ruptured membranes

ASSOCIATED RISKS

- Scalp lacerations
- Subdural hematoma of the neonate
- Cephalohematoma
- Maternal lacerations to the cervix, vagina, or perineum

INDICATIONS

- Maternal exhaustion and ineffective pushing efforts
- Fetal distress during second stage of labor
- Generally not used to assist birth before 34 weeks gestation

CONSIDERATIONS

PREPARATION OF THE CLIENT

- Provide the client and partner with support and education regarding the procedure.
- Assist the client into the lithotomy position to allow for sufficient traction of the vacuum cup when it is applied to the fetal head.
- Monitor and record FHR before and during vacuum assistance.
- Check for bladder distention, and catheterize if necessary.

ONGOING CARE: Prepare for a forceps-assisted birth if a vacuum-assisted birth is not successful.

NURSING ACTIONS

- Alert postpartum care providers that vacuum assistance was used.
- Observe the neonate for lacerations, cephalohematomas, or subdural hematomas after delivery.
- Check the neonate for caput succedaneum (swelling of the scalp in a newborn that usually disappears within 3 to 5 days).

Forceps-assisted birth

A forceps-assisted birth consists of using an instrument with two curved spoon-like blades to assist in the delivery of the fetal head. Traction is applied during contractions.

INDICATIONS

CLIENT PRESENTATION

- Prolonged second stage of labor and need to shorten duration (maternal exhaustion)
- Fetal distress during labor
- Abnormal presentation or a breech position requiring delivery of the head
- Arrest of rotation

CONSIDERATIONS

PREPARATION OF THE CLIENT

- Explain the procedure to the client and her partner.
- Assist the client into the lithotomy position.
- Ensure that the client's bladder is empty. Catheterize if necessary.
- The fetus must be engaged and the membranes ruptured.

INTERVENTIONS

- Monitor and record FHR before, during, and after forceps assistance.
  - Compression of the cord between the fetal head and forceps will cause a decrease in the FHR.
  - If a FHR decrease occurs, the forceps are removed and reapplied.
- Observe the neonate for bruising and abrasions at the site of forceps application after birth.

- Check the client for any possible injuries after birth.
  - Vaginal or cervical lacerations indicated by bleeding in spite of contracted uterus
  - Urine retention resulting from bladder or urethral injuries
  - Hematoma formation in the pelvic soft tissues resulting from blood vessel damage
- Report to the postpartum nursing caregivers that forceps or vacuum-assisted delivery methods were used.

COMPLICATIONS

- Lacerations of the cervix
- Lacerations of the vagina and perineum
- Injury to the bladder
- Facial nerve palsy of the neonate
- Facial bruising on the neonate

Episiotomy

An episiotomy is an incision made into the perineum to enlarge the vaginal opening to facilitate birth and minimize soft tissue damage.

INDICATIONS

- Shorten the second stage of labor
- Facilitate forceps-or vacuum-assisted delivery
- Prevent cerebral hemorrhage in a fragile preterm fetus
- Facilitate birth of a macrosomic (large) infant

CONSIDERATIONS

The site and direction of the incision designates the type of episiotomy.
- **Median (midline) episiotomy** extends from the vaginal outlet toward the rectum. It is the most commonly used.
  - Effective
  - Easily repaired
  - Generally least painful
  - Associated with a higher incidence of third- and fourth-degree lacerations
- A **mediolateral episiotomy** extends from the vaginal outlet posterolateral, either to the left or right of the midline, and is used when posterior extension is likely.
  - Third-degree laceration can occur.
  - Blood loss is greater, and the repair is more difficult and painful.
  - Local anesthetic is administered to the perineum prior to the incision.

ONGOING CARE: Encourage alternate labor positions to reduce pressure on the perineum and promote perineal stretching to reduce the necessity for an episiotomy.

Cesarean birth

- A cesarean birth is the delivery of the fetus through a transabdominal incision of the uterus to preserve the life or health of the client and fetus when there is evidence of complications.
- Incisions are made horizontally into the lower segment of the uterus.

INDICATIONS

POTENTIAL DIAGNOSES
- Malpresentation, particularly breech presentation
- Cephalopelvic disproportion
- Nonreassuring fetal heart tones
- Placental abnormalities
- Placenta previa
- Abruptio placentae
- High-risk pregnancy
  - Positive HIV status
  - Hypertensive disorders (preeclampsia, eclampsia)
  - Diabetes mellitus
  - Active genital herpes lesions
- Previous cesarean birth
- Dystocia
- Multiple gestations
- Umbilical cord prolapse

CONSIDERATIONS

PREPROCEDURE

NURSING ACTIONS
- Monitor and record FHR and vital signs.
- Position the client in a supine position with a wedge under one hip to prevent compression of the vena cava.
- Insert an indwelling urinary catheter.
- Ensure informed consent is obtained.
- Apply a sequential compression device.
- Administer preoperative medications.
- Prepare the surgical site.
- Assist in the insertion of an IV catheter, and ensure administration of IV fluids.
- Determine whether the client has had nothing by mouth since midnight before the procedure. If the client has, notify the anesthesiologist.
- Ensure that preoperative diagnostic tests are complete, including an Rh-factor test.
- Provide emotional support.

POSTPROCEDURE

- Monitor for evidence of infection and excessive bleeding at the incision site.
- Check the uterine fundus for firmness or tenderness.
- Check the lochia for amount and characteristics.

  A tender uterus and foul-smelling lochia can indicate endometritis.

- Monitor for productive cough or chills, which could be a manifestation of pneumonia.

- Check for indications of thrombophlebitis (tenderness, pain, heat on palpation).
- Monitor I&O.
- Monitor vital signs per protocol.
- Provide pain relief and antiemetics.
- Encourage the client to turn, cough, and deep breathe to prevent pulmonary complications.
- Encourage splinting of the incision with pillows.
- Encourage ambulation to prevent thrombus formation.
- Monitor the client for burning and pain on urination, which could be suggestive of a urinary tract infection.

COMPLICATIONS

MATERNAL
- Aspiration
- Amniotic fluid pulmonary embolism
- Wound infection
- Wound dehiscence
- Severe abdominal pain
- Thrombophlebitis
- Hemorrhage
- Urinary tract infection
- Injuries to the bladder or bowel
- Anesthesia associated complications

FETAL
- Premature birth of fetus if gestational age is inaccurate
- Fetal injuries during surgery

Complications Related to the Labor Process

Complications occurring during the labor process are emergent and require immediate intervention in order to improve maternal fetal outcomes.

Prolapsed umbilical cord

A prolapsed umbilical cord occurs when the umbilical cord is displaced, preceding the presenting part of the fetus, or protruding through the cervix. This results in cord compression and compromised fetal circulation. (10.5)

DATA COLLECTION

RISK FACTORS

- Rupture of amniotic membranes
- Abnormal fetal presentation (any presentation other than vertex [occiput as presenting part])
- Transverse lie: Presenting part is not engaged, which leaves room for the cord to descend.
- Small-for-gestational-age fetus
- Unusually long umbilical cord
- Multifetal pregnancy
- Unengaged presenting part
- Hydramnios or polyhydramnios

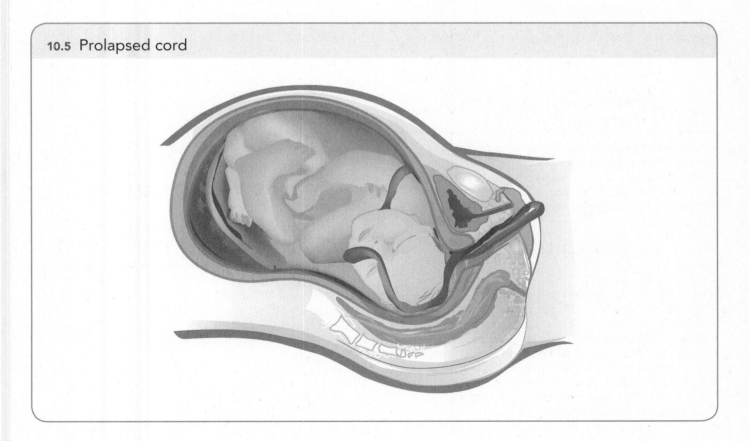

10.5 Prolapsed cord

EXPECTED FINDINGS

Client reports that she feels something coming through the vagina.

PHYSICAL FINDINGS

- Visualization or palpation of the umbilical cord protruding from the introitus
- FHR monitoring shows variable or prolonged deceleration
- Excessive fetal activity followed by cessation of movement; suggestive of severe fetal hypoxia

PATIENT-CENTERED CARE

NURSING CARE

- Call for assistance immediately.
- Notify the provider.
- The provider or RN will use a sterile-gloved hand, insert two fingers into the vagina, and apply finger pressure on either side of the cord to the fetal presenting part to elevate it off of the cord. Qs
- Reposition the client in a knee-chest, Trendelenburg, or a side-lying position with a rolled towel under the client's right or left hip to relieve pressure on the cord. QEBP
- Apply a warm, sterile, saline-soaked towel to the visible cord to prevent drying and to maintain blood flow.
- Provide continuous electronic monitoring of FHR for variable decelerations, which indicate fetal asphyxia and hypoxia.
- Administer oxygen at 8 to 10 L/min via a face mask to improve fetal oxygenation.
- Assist in initiating IV access and administering IV fluid bolus.
- Prepare for an immediate vaginal birth if cervix is fully dilated or cesarean section if it is not.
- Inform and educate the client and her partner about the interventions.

Meconium-stained amniotic fluid

- Meconium passage in the amniotic fluid during the antepartum period prior to the start of labor is typically not associated with an unfavorable fetal outcome.
- The fetus has had an episode of loss of sphincter control, allowing meconium to pass into amniotic fluid.

DATA COLLECTION

RISK FACTORS

- There is an increased incidence for meconium in the amniotic fluid after 38 weeks of gestation due to fetal maturity of normal physiological functions.
- Umbilical cord compression results in fetal hypoxia that stimulates the vagal nerve in mature fetuses.
- Hypoxia stimulates the vagal nerve, which induces peristalsis of the fetal gastrointestinal tract and relaxation of the anal sphincter.

EXPECTED FINDINGS

PHYSICAL FINDINGS

Amniotic fluid can vary in color (black to greenish, yellow, or brown), though meconium-stained amniotic fluid is often green. Consistency can be thin or thick.

Criteria for evaluation of meconium-stained amniotic fluid

- Often present in breech presentation, and might not indicate fetal hypoxia
- Present with no changes in FHR
- Stained fluid accompanied by variable or late decelerations in FHR (ominous sign)

DIAGNOSTIC PROCEDURES

Electronic fetal monitoring

PATIENT-CENTERED CARE

NURSING CARE

- Document color and consistency of stained amniotic fluid.
- Notify neonatal resuscitation team to be present at birth.

Fetal distress

Fetal distress is present when
- FHR is below 110/min or above 160/min.
- FHR shows decreased or no variability.
- There is fetal hyperactivity or no fetal activity.

EXPECTED FINDINGS: Nonreassuring FHR pattern with decreased or no variability

DIAGNOSTIC PROCEDURES
- Monitor uterine contractions.
- Monitor FHR.
- Monitor findings of ultrasound and other diagnostics.

RISK FACTORS
- Fetal anomalies
- Uterine anomalies
- Complications of labor and birth

PATIENT-CENTERED CARE

NURSING CARE

- Monitor vital signs and FHR.
- Position the client in a left side-lying reclining position with legs elevated.
- Administer 8 to 10 L/min of oxygen via a face mask.
- Oxytocin should be discontinued.
- Increase IV fluid rate to treat hypotension if indicated.
- Prepare the client for an emergency cesarean birth.

Application Exercises

1. A nurse in the labor and delivery unit is assisting with the care of a client in labor and applies an external fetal monitor and tocotransducer. The FHR is around 140/min. Contractions are occurring every 8 min and 30 to 40 seconds in duration. The RN performs a vaginal exam and finds the cervix is 2 cm dilated and 50% effaced, and the fetus is at a -2 station. Which of the following stages and phases of labor is this client experiencing?

   A. First stage, latent phase

   B. First stage, active phase

   C. First stage, transition phase

   D. Second stage of labor

2. A client experiences a large gush of fluid from her vagina while walking in the hallway of the birthing unit. Which of the following actions should the nurse take first?

   A. Check the amniotic fluid for meconium.

   B. Monitor FHR for distress.

   C. Dry the client and make her comfortable.

   D. Monitor uterine contractions.

3. A nurse is assisting with the care of a client who is at 40 weeks of gestation and experiencing contractions every 3 to 5 min and becoming stronger. A vaginal exam reveals that the client's cervix is 3 cm dilated, 80% effaced, and -1 station. The client asks for pain medication. Which of the following actions should the nurse take? (Select all that apply.)

   A. Encourage use of patterned breathing techniques.

   B. Insert an indwelling urinary catheter.

   C. Administer opioid analgesic medication.

   D. Suggest application of cold.

   E. Provide ice chips.

4. A nurse is caring for a client who has been in labor for 12 hr, and her membranes are intact. The provider has decided to perform an amniotomy in an effort to facilitate the progress of labor. The nurse performs a vaginal examination to ensure which of the following prior to the performance of the amniotomy?

   A. Fetal engagement

   B. Fetal lie

   C. Fetal attitude

   D. Fetal position

5. A nurse is assisting with the care of a client in active labor. When last examined 2 hr ago, the client's cervix was 3 cm dilated, 100% effaced, membranes intact, and the fetus was at a -2 station. The client suddenly states her water broke. The monitor reveals a FHR of 80 to 85/min. The nurse observes clear fluid and a loop of pulsating umbilical cord outside the client's vagina. Which of the following actions should the nurse perform first?

   A. Place the client in the Trendelenburg position.

   B. Apply finger pressure to the presenting part.

   C. Administer oxygen at 10 L/min via a face mask.

   D. Call for assistance.

PRACTICE Active Learning Scenario

A nurse is contributing to the plan of care for a client who experienced a cesarean birth. What should the nurse include in the plan of care? Use the ATI Active Learning Template: Therapeutic Procedure to complete this item.

DESCRIPTION OF PROCEDURE

INDICATIONS: Describe at least four.

NURSING INTERVENTIONS: Describe four that are preprocedure.

POTENTIAL COMPLICATIONS: Describe two that are maternal and two that are fetal.

Application Exercises Key

1. A. **CORRECT:** In stage 1, latent phase, the cervix dilates from 0 to 3 cm, and contraction duration ranges from 30 to 45 seconds.

   B. In stage 1, active phase, the cervix dilates from 4 to 7 cm, and contraction duration ranges from 40 to 70 seconds.

   C. In stage 1, transition phase, the cervix dilates from 8 to 10 cm, and contraction duration ranges from 45 to 90 seconds.

   D. The second stage of labor consists of the expulsion of the fetus.

   Ⓝ *NCLEX® Connection: Health Promotion and Maintenance, Ante/Intra/Postpartum and Newborn Care*

2. A. The nurse checks the color, clarity, odor, and amount of amniotic fluid, but this is not the first action the nurse should take.

   B. **CORRECT:** The greatest risk to the client and fetus is umbilical cord prolapse, leading to fetal distress following rupture of membranes. The first action by the nurse is to monitor the FHR for manifestations of distress.

   C. The nurse should provide comfort by drying the client following rupture of the membranes, but this is not the first action the nurse should take.

   D. The nurse monitors uterine contraction pattern after rupture of membranes, but this is not the first action the nurse should take.

   Ⓝ *NCLEX® Connection: Physiological Adaptation, Unexpected Response to Therapies*

3. A. **CORRECT:** Patterned breathing techniques can assist with pain management at this time.

   B. There is no indication for the insertion of an indwelling urinary catheter at this time.

   C. **CORRECT:** An opioid analgesic can be safely administered at this time.

   D. **CORRECT:** A nonpharmacological approach, such as the application of cold, is an appropriate intervention at this time.

   E. This action does not address the client's request for assistance with pain management.

   Ⓝ *NCLEX® Connection: Basic Care and Comfort, Nonpharmacological Comfort Interventions*

4. A. **CORRECT:** Prior to an amniotomy, it is imperative that the fetus is engaged at 0 station and at the level of the maternal ischial spines to prevent prolapse of the umbilical cord.

   B. Fetal lie pertains to the axis of the maternal spine in relation to the fetal spine and is determined by Leopold maneuvers.

   C. Fetal attitude is the relationship of the fetal extremities and chin to the fetal torso. It is determined by Leopold maneuvers.

   D. Fetal position refers to the direction of a reference point in the fetal presenting part to the maternal pelvis. It is not a criterion when performing an amniotomy.

   Ⓝ *NCLEX® Connection: Health Promotion and Maintenance, Ante/Intra/Postpartum and Newborn Care*

5. A. The nurse should place the client in the Trendelenburg position. However, another action is the priority.

   B. The nurse should apply pressure to the presenting part with her fingers. However, another action is the priority.

   C. The nurse should administer oxygen at 10 L/min via a face mask. However, another action is the priority.

   D. **CORRECT:** According to evidence-based practice, the nurse should first call for assistance.

   Ⓝ *NCLEX® Connection: Physiological Adaptation, Unexpected Response to Therapies*

PRACTICE Answer

Using the ATI Active Learning Template: Therapeutic Procedure

DESCRIPTION OF PROCEDURE:
Delivery of the fetus through a transabdominal incision of the uterus to preserve the life or health of the client and fetus when there is evidence of complications. Incisions are made horizontally into the lower uterine segment.

INDICATIONS
- Malpresentation, breech
- Cephalopelvic disproportion
- Fetal distress
- Placenta previa
- Abruptio placentae
- HIV-positive status
- Dystocia
- Multiple gestations
- Umbilical cord prolapse
- Preeclampsia
- Eclampsia
- Active herpes lesions
- Previous cesarean birth

NURSING INTERVENTIONS
- Monitor and record fetal heart rate and vital signs.
- Assist with ultrasound.
- Position client in a supine position with a wedge under one hip.
- Insert an indwelling urinary catheter.
- Administer preoperative medication.
- Prepare the surgical site.
- Assist in inserting an IV catheter and administering IV fluids.
- Ensure signed informed consent form is obtained.
- Determine NPO status.
- Verify preoperative testing results.
- Provide emotional support.

POTENTIAL COMPLICATIONS
- Maternal
  - Aspiration
  - Amniotic fluid pulmonary embolism
  - Wound infection
  - Wound dehiscence
  - Severe abdominal pain
  - Thrombophlebitis
  - Hemorrhage
  - Urinary tract infection
  - Injury to bladder or bowel
  - Anesthesia-associated complications
- Fetal
  - Premature birth
  - Fetal injury during surgery

Ⓝ *NCLEX® Connection: Health Promotion and Maintenance, Ante/Intra/Postpartum and Newborn Care*

UNIT 2   INTRAPARTUM NURSING CARE

CHAPTER 11   # Fetal Monitoring During Labor

Diagnostic procedures for fetal monitoring during labor include intermittent auscultation of the fetal heart rate (FHR) and palpation of uterine contractions, and internal monitoring of the FHR and uterine contractions.

Intermittent auscultation and uterine contraction palpation

Intermittent auscultation of the FHR is a low-technology method that can be performed during labor using a handheld Doppler ultrasound device, ultrasound stethoscope, or fetoscope to monitor FHR. In conjunction, palpation of contractions at the fundus for frequency, intensity, duration, and resting tone is used to evaluate fetal well-being. During labor, uterine contractions compress the uteroplacental arteries, temporarily stopping maternal blood flow into the uterus and intervillous spaces of the placenta, decreasing fetal circulation and oxygenation. Circulation to the uterus and placenta resumes during uterine relaxation between contractions. For low-risk labor and delivery, intermittent auscultation and palpation allows the client freedom of movement and can be done at home or a birthing center.

Guidelines for intermittent auscultation or continuous electronic fetal monitoring
- During latent phase: every 30 to 60 min
- During active phase: every 15 to 30 min
- During second stage: every 5 to 15 min

INDICATIONS

- Following rupture of membranes, spontaneously or artificially
- Preceding and subsequent to ambulation
- Prior to and following administration of or a change in medication or analgesia
- At time of expected peak action of anesthesia
- Following vaginal examination
- After urinary catheterization
- During abnormal or excessive uterine contractions

CONSIDERATIONS

PREPARATION OF THE CLIENT
- Monitor uterine activity.
- Palpate the uterine fundus to determine the size, lie, and presentation of the fetus.
- Place Doppler or other device over area of maximal intensity to auscultate FHR.
- Count FHR for 30 to 60 seconds between contractions to determine baseline rate.
- Auscultate FHR before, during, and after a contraction to determine FHR in response to the contractions.

ONGOING CARE: Identify FHR patterns and characteristics of uterine contractions.

NURSING ACTIONS
- Monitor the FHR and characteristics of uterine contractions, implement nursing interventions, and report a nonreassuring FHR or abnormal uterine contractions to the RN, nurse practitioner, midwife, or provider.
- Cultural considerations, as well as the emotional, educational, and comfort needs of the mother and the family, must be incorporated into the plan of care while continuing to monitor the FHR response to uterine contractions during the labor process. Qᴘᴄᴄ

> The method and frequency of fetal surveillance during labor varies and depends on maternal/fetal risk factors as well as the preference of the facility, provider, and client.

INTERPRETATION OF FINDINGS

- A reassuring FHR is 110 to 160/min with increases and decreases from baseline.
- Tachycardia is a FHR greater than 160/min for 1 min or longer.
- Bradycardia is a FHR less than 110/min for 1 min or longer.

Continuous electronic fetal monitoring

Continuous external fetal monitoring is accomplished by securing an ultrasound transducer over the abdomen to record the FHR pattern, and a tocotransducer on the fundus to record the uterine contractions.

ADVANTAGES
- Noninvasive and reduces risk for infection.
- Membranes do not have to be ruptured.
- Cervix does not have to be dilated.
- Placement of transducers can be performed by the nurse.
- Provides permanent record of FHR and uterine contraction tracing.

DISADVANTAGES
- Contraction intensity is not measurable.
- Movement of the client requires frequent repositioning of transducers.
- Quality of recording is affected by client weight and fetal position.

CONSIDERATIONS

PREPARATION OF THE CLIENT
- Place ultrasound transducer over area of maximal intensity to auscultate FHR.
- Palpate the fundus to determine proper placement of the tocotransducer.

ONGOING CARE
- Reinforce education regarding the procedure to the client and the client's partner during placement and adjustments of the fetal monitor equipment. Explain the purpose and reassure the client that use of monitoring does not imply fetal jeopardy.
- Encourage the client to make frequent position changes, which will require adjustments of the transducers.
- If the client needs to void and it is not contraindicated, the nurse can disconnect the external monitor temporarily.
- If disconnecting the FHR monitor is contraindicated or an internal FHR monitor is being used, the nurse can bring the client a bedpan.

INTERPRETATION OF FINDINGS

- An expected baseline fetal heart rate at term is 110 to 160/min. This is excluding accelerations, decelerations, and periods of marked variability within a 10 min window. At least 2 min of baseline segments in 10 min should be present. A single number should be documented instead of a baseline range.
- Fetal heart rate baseline variability is described as fluctuations in the FHR baseline that are irregular in frequency and amplitude. Expected variability should be moderate variability.
- Changes in fetal heart rate patterns are categorized as episodic or periodic changes. Episodic changes are not associated with uterine contractions, and periodic changes occur with uterine contractions. These changes include accelerations and decelerations.

- Interpretation of FHR patterns is the responsibility of the RN, nurse practitioner, midwife, or provider.
- Each uterine contraction is comprised of the following.
  - **Increment:** the beginning of the contraction as intensity is increasing
  - **Acme:** the peak intensity of the contraction
  - **Decrement:** the decline of the contraction intensity as the contraction is ending

FHR PATTERNS

Accelerations

Variable transitory increase in the FHR above baseline

CAUSES/COMPLICATIONS
- Healthy fetal/placental exchange
- Intact fetal central nervous system (CNS) response to fetal movement
- Vaginal exam
- Uterine contractions
- Fundal pressure

SIGNIFICANCE
- Characteristic pattern
- Occurs with fetal movement
- Indicates fetal welfare (state of arousal/alertness)

Fetal bradycardia

FHR less than 110/min for 10 min or more

CAUSES/COMPLICATIONS
- Uteroplacental insufficiency
- Umbilical cord prolapse
- Maternal hypotension
- Prolonged umbilical cord compression
- Fetal congenital heart block
- Anesthetic medications
- Viral infection
- Maternal hypoglycemia
- Fetal heart failure
- Maternal hypothermia

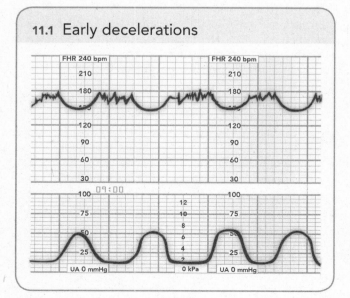

11.1 Early decelerations

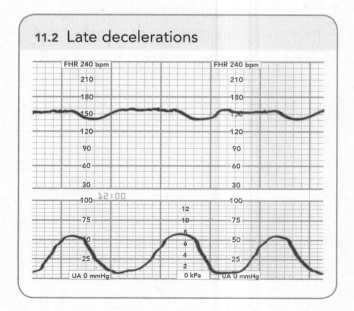

11.2 Late decelerations

NURSING ACTIONS

- Discontinue oxytocin if being administered.
- Assist the client to a side-lying position.
- Administer oxygen at 10 L/min via nonrebreather face mask.
- Monitor maintenance IV fluids.
- Administer a tocolytic medication.
- Notify the provider.

Fetal tachycardia

FHR greater than 160/min for 10 min or more

CAUSES/COMPLICATIONS
- Maternal infection, fever, chorioamnionitis
- Fetal anemia
- Fetal cardiac dysrhythmias
- Maternal use of cocaine or methamphetamines
- Maternal dehydration
- Maternal hyperthyroidism

NURSING ACTIONS
- Administer antipyretics for maternal fever.
- Administer oxygen at 10 L/min via nonrebreather face mask.
- Monitor IV fluid bolus.

Early deceleration of FHR

Slowing of the FHR at the beginning of a contraction with the return of the FHR to baseline at the end of a contraction

CAUSES/COMPLICATIONS
- Compression of the fetal head resulting from uterine contraction
- Uterine contractions
- Vaginal exam
- Fundal pressure

Late deceleration of FHR

Slowing of FHR after contraction has started with return of FHR to baseline well after contraction has ended

CAUSES/COMPLICATIONS
- Uteroplacental insufficiency causing inadequate fetal oxygenation
- Maternal hypotension, placenta previa, abruptio placentae, uterine tachysystole
- Preeclampsia
- Late- or post-term pregnancy
- Maternal diabetes mellitus

NURSING ACTIONS
- Place client in side-lying position.
- Increase rate of IV maintenance solution.
- Discontinue oxytocin if being infused.
- Administer oxygen at 8 to 10 L/min via nonrebreather face mask.
- Correct hypotension by elevating the client's legs.
- Notify the provider.
- Assist with placement of an internal monitor.
- Prepare for vaginal or cesarean birth if there is no change in pattern.

Variable deceleration of FHR

Transitory, abrupt slowing of FHR less than 110/min, variable in duration, intensity, and timing in relation to uterine contraction

CAUSES/COMPLICATIONS
- Umbilical cord compression
- Short cord
- Prolapsed cord
- Nuchal cord (around fetal neck)

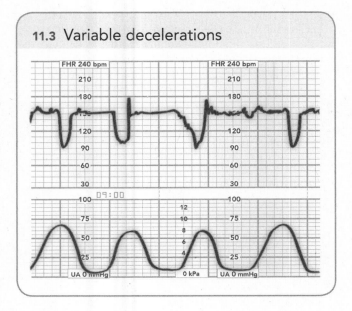

11.3 Variable decelerations

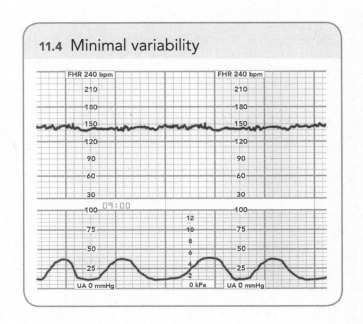

11.4 Minimal variability

NURSING ACTIONS

- Place client in side-lying or knee-chest position.
- Discontinue oxytocin if being infused.
- Administer oxygen at 8 to 10 L/min via nonrebreather face mask.
- Notify the provider.
- Assist with a vaginal examination to identify prolapsed cord.
- Assist with an amnioinfusion if necessary.
- Prepare for vaginal or cesarean birth.

Continuous internal fetal monitoring

Continuous internal fetal monitoring with a scalp electrode is performed by attaching a small spiral electrode to the presenting part of the fetus to monitor the FHR. The electrode wires are then attached to a leg plate that is placed on the thigh and then attached to the fetal monitor.

INDICATIONS

Continuous internal fetal monitoring can be used in conjunction with an intrauterine pressure catheter (IUPC), which is a solid or fluid-filled transducer placed inside the client's uterine cavity to monitor the frequency, duration, and intensity of contractions. The average pressure is usually 50 to 85 mm Hg.

ADVANTAGES

- Early detection of abnormal FHR patterns can be suggestive of fetal distress
- Accurate data collection of FHR variability
- Accurate measurement of uterine contraction intensity
- Allows greater maternal freedom of movement because tracing is not affected by fetal activity, maternal position changes, or weight

DISADVANTAGES

- Membranes must have ruptured to use internal monitoring.
- Cervix must be dilated a minimum of 2 to 3 cm.
- Presenting part must have descended enough for proper electrode placement.
- A provider, nurse practitioner, midwife, or specifically trained RN must perform this procedure.

CONSIDERATIONS

PREPARATION OF THE CLIENT

- Ensure electronic fetal monitoring equipment is functioning properly.
- Use aseptic techniques when assisting with procedures.

ONGOING CARE

- Monitor maternal vital signs, and obtain maternal temperature every 1 to 2 hr.
- Encourage the client to reposition frequently. If the client is lying supine, place a wedge under one of the hips to tilt the uterus.

Leopold maneuvers

Leopold maneuvers consist of performing external palpations of the maternal uterus through the abdominal wall to determine the following.

- Number of fetuses
- Presenting part, fetal lie, and fetal attitude
- Degree of descent of the presenting part into the pelvis
- Location of the fetus's back to check fetal heart tones
  - **Vertex presentation:** Check fetal heart tones below the mother's umbilicus in either the right- or left-lower quadrant of the abdomen.
  - **Breech presentation:** Check fetal heart tones above the mother's umbilicus in either the right- or left-upper quadrant of the abdomen.

CONSIDERATIONS

PREPARATION OF THE CLIENT

- Ask the client to empty her bladder before the examination.
- Place the client in the supine position with a pillow under her head, and have her knees slightly flexed.
- Place a small, rolled towel under the client's right or left hip to displace the uterus off the major blood vessels to prevent supine hypotensive syndrome.

ONGOING CARE

- Identify the fetal part occupying the fundus. The head should feel round, firm, and move freely. The breech should feel irregular and soft. This maneuver identifies the fetal lie (longitudinal or transverse) and presenting part (cephalic or breech).
- Validate the presenting part. Locate and palpate the smooth contour of the fetal back using the palm of one hand and the irregular small parts of the hands, feet, and elbows using the palm of the other hand.
- Identify the descent of the presenting part into the pelvis. Determine the part that is presenting over the true pelvis inlet by gently grasping the lower segment of the uterus between the thumb and fingers. If the head is presenting and not engaged, determine whether the head is flexed or extended.
- Identify the fetal attitude. Face the client's feet and outline the fetal head using the palmar surface of the fingertips on both hands to palpate the cephalic prominence. If the cephalic prominence is on the same side as the small parts, the head is flexed with vertex presentation. If the cephalic prominence is on the same side as the back, the head is extended with a face presentation.

NURSING ACTIONS

- Auscultate the FHR post-maneuvers to determine fetal tolerance to the procedure.
- Document the findings from the maneuvers.

Application Exercises

1. A nurse is discussing intermittent fetal heart monitoring with a newly licensed nurse. Which of the following statements should the nurse include?

   A. "Count the fetal heart rate for 15 seconds to determine the baseline."

   B. "Auscultate the fetal heart rate immediately following rupture of membranes."

   C. "Count the fetal heart rate during a contraction to determine the baseline."

   D. "Auscultate the fetal heart rate every 30 minutes during the second stage of labor."

2. A nurse is reinforcing teaching with a client about the benefits of internal fetal heart monitoring. Which of the following statements should the nurse include? (Select all that apply.)

   A. "It is considered a noninvasive procedure."

   B. "It can detect abnormal fetal heart tones early."

   C. "It can determine the amount of amniotic fluid you have."

   D. "It allows for accurate readings despite maternal movement."

   E. "It can measure uterine contraction intensity."

3. A nurse is assisting in the care of a client who is in active labor. The nurse notes tachycardia on the external fetal monitor tracing. Which of the following conditions should the nurse identify as a potential cause of the heart rate?

   A. Maternal fever

   B. Fetal heart failure

   C. Maternal hypoglycemia

   D. Fetal head compression

4. A nurse is caring for a client who is in labor and is experiencing late decelerations in the FHR. Which of the following actions should the nurse take first?

   A. Assist the client into the left-lateral position.

   B. Apply oxygen at 10L/min via a nonrebreather face mask.

   C. Increase the rate of the maintenance IV fluid.

   D. Prepare the client for a vaginal exam.

5. A nurse is reinforcing teaching about external monitoring with a client who was recently admitted for induction of labor. Which of the following information should the nurse include?

   A. Membranes must be ruptured prior to monitor placement.

   B. There is an increased risk for infection when using an external monitor.

   C. External monitoring cannot measure intensity of contractions.

   D. The monitor must be applied by the provider or a nurse midwife.

PRACTICE Active Learning Scenario

A nurse is reviewing intermittent fetal auscultation and uterine contraction palpation with a newly licensed nurse. What information should the nurse include in the review? Use the ATI Active Learning Template: Therapeutic Procedure to complete this item.

INDICATIONS: Describe four situations when this procedure should be performed.

OUTCOMES/EVALUATION: Describe expected FHR findings.

NURSING INTERVENTIONS
- Preprocedure: Describe the three types of devices that are used to monitor FHR.
- Intraprocedure: Identify the time frame for counting FHR to determine the baseline rate and when auscultation should take place.

1. A. The nurse should count the FHR for 30 to 60 seconds to determine the baseline.

   B. **CORRECT:** The nurse should auscultate the FHR immediately following rupture of membranes to monitor for changes that can indicate umbilical cord prolapse.

   C. The nurse should count the FHR between contractions to determine the baseline.

   D. The nurse should auscultate the FHR every 5 to 15 min during the second stage of labor.

   (N) NCLEX® Connection: Health Promotion and Maintenance, Ante/ Intra/Postpartum and Newborn Care

2. A. A disadvantage of internal fetal monitoring is that it is an invasive procedure.

   B. **CORRECT:** A benefit of internal fetal monitoring is that it can detect abnormal fetal heart tones early.

   C. Internal fetal monitoring cannot determine the amount of amniotic fluid.

   D. **CORRECT:** A benefit of internal fetal monitoring is that it allows for accurate readings despite maternal movement; external monitoring requires adjustment when the client moves.

   E. **CORRECT:** A benefit of internal fetal monitoring is that it can measure uterine contraction intensity; external monitoring cannot.

   (N) NCLEX® Connection: Reduction of Risk Potential, Diagnostic Tests

3. A. **CORRECT:** Tachycardia can be caused by maternal fever, infection, and chorioamnionitis.

   B. Fetal heart failure can cause bradycardia in the FHR.

   C. Maternal hypoglycemia can cause bradycardia in the FHR.

   D. Fetal head compression can cause early decelerations in the FHR.

   (N) NCLEX® Connection: Reduction of Risk Potential, Potential for Alterations in Body Systems

4. A. **CORRECT:** The greatest risk to the fetus during late decelerations is uteroplacental insufficiency. The first action the nurse should take is place the client into the left-lateral position to increase uteroplacental perfusion.

   B. The nurse should apply oxygen at 10L/min via nonrebreather face mask to increase fetal oxygenation. However, there is another action the nurse should take first.

   C. The nurse should increase the rate of the maintenance IV fluid to increase hydration and enhance placental perfusion. However, there is another action the nurse should take first.

   D. The nurse should prepare the client for a vaginal exam performed by the nurse or provider to determine cervical dilation. However, there is another action the nurse should take first.

   (N) NCLEX® Connection: Physiological Adaptation, Alterations in Body Systems

5. A. External monitoring can be used whether the membranes are ruptured or intact.

   B. Internal monitoring increases the risk for infection.

   C. **CORRECT:** An intrauterine pressure catheter measures the intensity of uterine contractions.

   D. External monitors can be applied by a nurse; an internal FHR monitor can be applied by a specifically trained RN, a nurse practitioner, midwife, or a provider. An IUPC can be inserted by a nurse practitioner/midwife or provider.

   (N) NCLEX® Connection: Reduction of Risk Potential, Diagnostic Tests

PRACTICE Answer

Using the ATI Active Learning Template: Therapeutic Procedure

INDICATIONS
- Determining active labor
- Rupture of membranes, spontaneously or artificially
- Preceding and subsequent to ambulation
- Prior to and following administration of or a change in medication analgesia
- At the peak action of anesthesia
- Following vaginal examination
- Following expulsion of an enema
- After urinary catheterization
- Abnormal or excessive uterine contractions

OUTCOMES/EVALUATION: A normal, reassuring FHR is 110 to 160/min with increases and decreases from baseline.

NURSING INTERVENTIONS
- Preprocedure
  - Handheld Doppler ultrasound
  - Ultrasound stethoscope
  - Fetoscope
- Intraprocedure
  - Count FHR for 30 to 60 seconds between contractions to determine baseline rate.
  - Auscultate FHR before, during, and after a contraction to determine FHR in response to the contractions.

(N) NCLEX® Connection: Reduction of Risk Potential, Diagnostic Tests

When reviewing the following chapters, keep in mind the relevant topics and tasks of the NCLEX outline, in particular:

Health Promotion and Maintenance

ANTE/INTRA/POSTPARTUM AND NEWBORN CARE
Perform care of postpartum client (perineal care, assistance with infant feeding).

Monitor recovery of stable postpartum client.

DATA COLLECTION TECHNIQUES: Collect baseline physical data (skin integrity, height and weight).

DEVELOPMENTAL STAGES AND TRANSITIONS: Assist client with expected life transition (attachment to newborn, parenting, retirement).

Pharmacological Therapies

EXPECTED ACTIONS/OUTCOMES: Apply knowledge of pathophysiology when addressing client pharmacological agents.

Physiological Adaptation

ALTERATIONS IN BODY SYSTEMS
Identify signs and symptoms of an infection (temperature changes, swelling, redness, mental confusion, foul smelling urine).

Provide care for a client experiencing complications of pregnancy/labor and/or delivery (eclampsia, precipitous labor, hemorrhage).

CHAPTER 12

CHAPTER 12 *Nursing Care of the Client During the Postpartum Period*

It is important to provide comfort measures for the client during the postpartum period, also called the fourth trimester of pregnancy. This maternal recovery period starts with delivery of the placenta and includes at least the first 2 hr after birth. During this stage, parent-newborn bonding should begin to occur.

The main goal during the immediate postpartum period is to monitor for postpartum hemorrhage. Other goals include assisting in recovery by recognizing and reporting irregularities in the expected healing process and providing comfort measures. The nurse should reinforce client education about newborn and self-care, and assist with providing baby-friendly activities to promote newborn/family bonding.

Discharge teaching is also an important aspect of postpartum care. A client should be able to perform self-care and recognize effects that suggest complications prior to discharge.

Discharge planning should be initiated at admission with time spent during the hospitalization on reinforcing postpartum self-care. A nurse should use a variety of strategies to promote learning. Return demonstrations are important to ensure that adequate learning has taken place.

DETERMINING A CLIENT'S KNOWLEDGE OF POSTPARTUM CARE

- Inquire about the client's knowledge regarding self-care.
- Determine the client's home support system and who will be present to assist. Include support persons in the educational process.
- Determine the client's readiness for learning and ability to verbalize or demonstrate the information given.

PHYSICAL CHANGES

The postpartum period, also known as the puerperium, includes physiological and psychological adjustments. This period is the interval between birth and the return of the reproductive organs to their normal nonpregnant state. Although traditionally this has been considered to last 6 weeks, the time frame varies.

- Physiological maternal changes consist of uterine involution; lochia flow; cervical involution; decrease in vaginal distention; alteration in ovarian function and menstruation; and cardiovascular, urinary tract, breast, and gastrointestinal tract changes.
- The greatest risks during the postpartum period are hemorrhage, shock, and infection.
- Oxytocin, a hormone released from the pituitary gland, coordinates and strengthens uterine contractions.
  - Breastfeeding stimulates the release of endogenous oxytocin from the pituitary gland.
  - Exogenous oxytocin can be administered postpartum to improve the quality of the uterine contractions. A firm and contracted uterus prevents excessive bleeding and hemorrhage.
  - Uncomfortable uterine cramping is referred to as afterpains.
- After delivery of the placenta, hormones (estrogen, progesterone, placental enzyme insulinase) decrease, resulting in decreased blood glucose, estrogen, and progesterone levels.
  - Decreased estrogen is associated with breast engorgement, diaphoresis (profuse perspiration), and diuresis (increased formation and excretion of urine) of excess extracellular fluid accumulated during pregnancy.
  - Decreased estrogen diminishes vaginal lubrication. Local dryness and discomfort during intercourse can persist until ovarian function returns and menstruation resumes.
  - Decreased progesterone results in an increase in muscle tone throughout the body.
  - Decreased placental enzyme insulinase results in reversal of the diabetogenic effects of pregnancy, which lowers blood glucose levels immediately in the puerperium.

DATA COLLECTION

Data collection in the immediate postpartum period includes monitoring vital signs, uterine firmness and location in relation to the umbilicus, uterine position in relation to the midline of the abdomen, and the amount of vaginal bleeding.

American Academy of Pediatrics and American Congress of Obstetricians and Gynecologists recommend blood pressure and pulse be checked at least every 15 min for the first 2 hr after birth. Temperature should be checked every 4 hr for the first 8 hr after birth and then at least every 8 hr.

Fundus

Physical changes of the uterus include involution. Involution occurs with contractions of the uterine smooth muscle, whereby the uterus returns to its prepregnant state. The uterus also rapidly decreases in size from approximately 1 kg (2.2 lb) to 60 to 80 g at 6 weeks with the fundal height steadily descending into the pelvis approximately one fingerbreadth (1 cm) per day. **(12.1)**

- Immediately after delivery, the fundus should be firm, midline with the umbilicus, and approximately at the level of the umbilicus. At 12 hr postpartum, the fundus can be palpated at 1 cm above the umbilicus.
- Every 24 hr, the fundus should descend approximately 1 to 2 cm. It should be halfway between the symphysis pubis and the umbilicus by the sixth postpartum day.
- After 2 weeks, the uterus should lie within the true pelvis and should not be palpable.

12.1 Fundal height

DATA COLLECTION

The nurse should assist with determining the fundal height, uterine placement, and uterine consistency at least every 8 hr after the recovery period has ended.

- Explain the procedure to the client.
- Apply clean gloves and a lower perineal pad, and observe lochia flow as the fundus is palpated.
- Cup one hand just above the symphysis pubis to support the lower segment of the uterus. With the other hand, palpate the abdomen to locate the fundus.
- Document the fundal height, location, and uterine consistency.
  - Determine the fundal height by placing fingers on the abdomen and measuring how many fingerbreadths (centimeters) fit between the fundus and the umbilicus above, below, or at the umbilical level.
  - Determine whether the fundus is midline in the pelvis or displaced laterally (caused by a full bladder).
  - Determine whether the fundus is firm or boggy. If the fundus is boggy (not firm), lightly massage the fundus in a circular motion. Q𝐄𝐁𝐏

PATIENT-CENTERED CARE

- Encourage early breastfeeding for a client who is lactating. Reinforce to the client that this will stimulate the production of natural oxytocin and prevent hemorrhage.
- Encourage emptying of the bladder every 2 to 3 hr. Reinforce to the client that this will prevent possible uterine displacement and loss of muscle tone.

Lochia

Lochia is post-birth uterine discharge that contains blood, mucus, and uterine tissue.

Three stages of lochia

Lochia rubra: Dark red to brown "period-like" discharge, containing debris from sloughing of the uterine lining. The flow lasts 1 to 3 days after delivery and increases with breastfeeding and ambulation. Remind the client that she might experience a surge of discharge upon arising after lying in bed for an extended period of time. This should not be mistaken for hemorrhage.

Lochia serosa: Pinkish brown, watery discharge, consisting of old blood, white blood cells, and debris from the uterine lining. The discharge lasts from approximately day 4 to day 10 after delivery.

Lochia alba: Yellowish or white creamy discharge consisting of serum, white blood cells, epithelial cells, and debris from the mucous membrane lining the uterus. This discharge lasts from approximately day 11 up to 8 weeks after delivery.

DATA COLLECTION

- Lochia amount is estimated by the quantity of saturation on the perineal pad.
  - Scant: less than 2.5 cm
  - Light: 2.5 to 10 cm
  - Moderate: more than 10 cm
  - Heavy: one pad saturated within 2 hr
  - Excessive blood loss: one pad saturated in 15 min or less, or the converging of blood under the buttocks. This is an indication of postpartum hemorrhage and should be reported to the charge nurse and provider immediately. (12.2) Qs
- Check the lochia flow for normal color, amount, and consistency.
  - Lochia typically trickles from the vaginal opening but flows more steadily during uterine contractions.
  - Check for pooled lochia on the pad under the client, which she might not feel. Massaging the uterus or ambulation can result in a gush of lochia with the expression of clots and dark blood that has pooled in the vagina, but should soon decrease back to a trickle of bright red lochia when in the early puerperium.

PATIENT-CENTERED CARE

Nursing interventions for abnormal lochia include notifying the charge nurse and provider as well as assisting with interventions based on the cause of the abnormality.

Recognizing manifestations of abnormal lochia

- Excessive spurting of bright red blood from the vagina, possibly indicating a cervical or vaginal tear
- Numerous large clots and excessive blood loss (saturation of one pad in 15 min or less), which can indicate hemorrhage
- Foul odor, which is suggestive of infection
- Persistent lochia rubra in the early postpartum period beyond day 3, which can indicate retained placental fragments
- Continued flow of lochia serosa or lochia alba beyond the normal length of time can indicate endometritis, especially if it is accompanied by fever, pain, or abdominal tenderness.

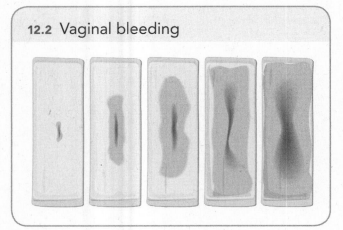

12.2 Vaginal bleeding

Cervix, vagina, and perineum

PHYSICAL CHANGES

- The cervix is soft directly after birth and can be edematous, bruised, and have small lacerations. Within 2 to 3 days postpartum, it shortens, regains its form, and becomes firm, with the cervical os gradually closing after being dilated to 10 cm during labor. Lacerations can delay the production of estrogen-influenced cervical mucus and are a predisposing factor to infection.
- The vagina, which has distended, gradually returns to its prepregnancy size with the reappearance of rugae and a thickening of the vaginal mucosa. However, muscle tone is never restored completely.
- The soft tissues of the perineum can appear red and swollen, especially in areas of an episiotomy or lacerations. Hematomas or hemorrhoids can be present. Pelvic floor muscles can be overstretched and weak.

Sexual intercourse

- Avoid sexual intercourse until the episiotomy/laceration is healed and vaginal discharge has turned white (lochia alba). This usually takes 2 to 4 weeks or until the client is seen by the provider. Over-the-counter lubricants might be needed during the first 6 weeks to 6 months.
- Physiological reactions to sexual activity can be slower and less intense for the first 3 months following birth.

Contraception

- Discuss the use of contraception upon resumption of sexual activity. Inform the client that pregnancy can occur while breastfeeding even though menses has not returned.
- Advise clients who are lactating that oral contraceptives should not be taken until milk production is well established (usually 4 weeks).
- Lactating and nonlactating women differ in the timing of the first ovulation and resumption of menstruation.
- Menses for nonlactating clients might not resume until around 4 to 10 weeks. However, ovulation can occur as early as 1 month after delivery.
- Menses for lactating clients might not resume for 3 months or until cessation of breastfeeding.
  - In lactating women, serum prolactin levels remain elevated and suppress ovulation.
    - The return of ovulation is influenced by breastfeeding frequency, length of each feeding, and use of supplementation.
    - The infant's suck is also believed to affect prolactin levels.
    - Length of time to the first postpartum ovulation is approximately 6 months.
    - In nonlactating clients, prolactin declines and reaches the prepregnant level by the third week postpartum. Ovulation occurs 27 to 75 days after birth.
    - Menses resumes by 4 to 6 weeks postpartum.

DATA COLLECTION

- Observe the perineum for redness, swelling, and the presence of a hematoma.
- Inspect episiotomy and lacerations for approximation, drainage, quantity, and quality. A bright red trickle of blood from the episiotomy site in the early postpartum period is an expected finding.

PATIENT-CENTERED CARE

Perineal tenderness, laceration, episiotomy

- Promote measures to help soften the client's stools.
- Reinforce education about proper cleansing to prevent infection.
  - Wash hands thoroughly before and after voiding.
  - Use a squeeze bottle filled with tap water warmed to 38° C (100.4° F) after each voiding to cleanse the perineal area.
  - Clean the perineal area from front to back (urethra to anus).
  - Blot dry; do not wipe.
  - Sparingly use a topical application of antiseptic cream or spray 3 to 4 times daily.
  - Change the perineal pad from front to back after voiding or defecating.
- Promote comfort measures.
  - Apply ice packs to the perineum consistently during the first 24 hr to reduce edema, and after the first 24 hr as desired to provide an analgesic effect.
  - Encourage sitz baths at a temperature of 40.6° C (105.1° F) or cooler at least twice a day for 20 minutes. Q̲EBP
  - Apply topical anesthetic cream or spray to the perineal area 3 to 4 times daily.
  - Apply witch hazel compresses to the perineum after voiding or defecating.
  - Apply hydrocortisone cream after cleansing to the external anal area for hemorrhoids.

Breasts

Physical changes of the breasts include the secretion of clear yellow fluid called colostrum, which occurs during pregnancy and 3 to 4 days immediately after birth. Milk is produced 72 to 96 hr after the birth of the newborn.

DATA COLLECTION

Check the client's breasts and ability to assist the newborn with latching on if breastfeeding. Ineffective newborn feeding patterns could be related to maternal dehydration, maternal discomfort, newborn positioning, or difficulty with the newborn latching onto the breast. Deviations from expected findings and complications with breastfeeding should be reported to the charge nurse.

- Inspect the client's breasts for the following
  - Redness and tenderness.
  - Cracked nipples and indications of mastitis (infection in a milk duct of the breast with concurrent flu-like manifestations).
- Colostrum (early milk) transitions to mature milk by about 72 to 96 hr after birth and is referred to as the "milk coming in."
- Engorgement of the breast tissue is a result of lymphatic circulation, milk production, and temporary vein congestion.

PATIENT-CENTERED CARE

- Encourage early demand breastfeeding for the client who is lactating. This will stimulate the production of natural oxytocin and help prevent uterine hemorrhage.
- Assist the client into a comfortable position, and reinforce teaching about the various positions during breastfeeding. The four traditional positions for breastfeeding are football hold (under the arm), cradle, across the lap (modified cradle), and side-lying. Reinforce how varying positions can prevent nipple soreness.
- Instruct the client about the importance of proper latch techniques (the newborn takes in part of the areola and nipple, not just the tip of the nipple) to prevent nipple soreness.
- Inform the client that breastfeeding causes the release of oxytocin, which stimulates uterine contractions. This is an expected occurrence and beneficial to uterine tone.

Cardiovascular system and fluid and hematologic status

PHYSICAL CHANGES

Cardiovascular system during the postpartum period
The cardiovascular system undergoes a decrease in blood volume during the postpartum period related to
- Blood loss during childbirth: Average blood loss is 300 to 500 mL (10% to 15% of blood volume) in an uncomplicated vaginal delivery and 500 to 1,000 mL (15% to 30% of blood volume) for a cesarean birth.
- Diaphoresis and diuresis of the excess fluid accumulated during the last part of the pregnancy. Loss occurs within the first 2 to 3 days postdelivery.

Nutrition

- Reinforce the importance of eating a nutritious diet including all food groups. A diet well-balanced in all key nutrients promotes healing and overall well-being in the postpartum period. Encourage a diet high in protein, which will aid in tissue repair. Remind the client to consume 2 to 3 L of fluid each day from food and beverage sources.
- Encourage moderately active, nonlactating clients to consume 1,800 to 2,200 kcal/day.
- Instruct lactating clients to increase caloric intake by 450 to 500 kcal/day and include calcium-enriched foods.
- Clients who are underweight or breastfeeding more than one infant require additional calorie intake.
- Lactating clients should incorporate 200 to 300 mg omega-3 polyunsaturated fatty acids in their diet to provide adequate DHA for the infant in the breast milk. Adding one or two portions of low-mercury fish to the diet will supply the additional DHA.
- Instruct clients who are vegan or malnourished to take multivitamin supplements and DHA.
- For clients who have decreased hemoglobin and hematocrit levels, iron supplements may be recommended.
- Remind the client that the use of prenatal vitamins may be prolonged until their current supply has been used or until 6 weeks postpartum.

Postpartum exercises

- Instruct the client how to regain pelvic floor muscle control by performing Kegel exercises. The same muscles are used when starting and stopping the flow of urine. Have the client rapidly contract and relax the pelvic floor muscles 10 to 25 times, three times per day.
- Reinforce teaching on how to perform pelvic tilt exercises to strengthen back muscles and relieve strain on the lower back. These exercises involve alternately arching and straightening the back.

VITAL SIGN CHANGES

- Blood pressure is temporarily increased by approximately 5% for the first few weeks after birth. Returning to prepregnancy levels may take weeks to months.
- Possible orthostatic hypotension within the first 48 hr postpartum can occur immediately after standing up with feelings of faintness or dizziness resulting from splanchnic (viscera/internal organs) engorgement that can occur after birth.
- Elevation of heart rate, stroke volume, and cardiac output for the first hour postpartum occurs and then gradually decreases to a prepregnant baseline during the next 48 hr.
- Elevation of temperature to 38° C (100.4° F) resulting from the dehydrating effects of labor during the first 24 hr can occur, but should return to prepregnancy levels after 24 hr postpartum.

DATA COLLECTION

- Check for cardiovascular and vital sign changes. Monitor blood component changes.
- Inspect the legs for redness, swelling, and warmth, which are additional indications of venous thrombosis.

PATIENT-CENTERED CARE

Nursing interventions for alterations in findings include notifying the charge nurse and provider, and performing interventions based on the cause of the alteration.
- Encourage early ambulation and apply antiembolism stockings to the lower extremities to prevent venous stasis and thrombosis.
- Remove the stockings as soon as the client is ambulating.
- Administer medications.

Gastrointestinal system and bowel function

EXPECTED PHYSICAL CHANGES IN THE GASTROINTESTINAL SYSTEM
- Increased appetite following delivery
- Constipation with bowel evacuation delayed until 2 to 3 days after birth
- Hemorrhoids

DATA COLLECTION

The nurse should check the gastrointestinal system including bowel function.
- Check for reports of hunger. Expect the client to have a good appetite.
- Check for bowel sounds and the return of expected bowel function. Spontaneous bowel movement might not occur for 2 to 3 days after delivery secondary to decreased intestinal muscle tone during labor and puerperium and prelabor diarrhea and dehydration. The client can also anticipate discomfort with defecation because of perineal tenderness, episiotomy, lacerations, or hemorrhoids.
- Check the rectal area for varicosities (hemorrhoids).
- Operative vaginal birth (forceps-and vacuum-assisted) and anal sphincter lacerations increase the risk of temporary postpartum anal incontinence that usually resolves within 6 months.

PATIENT-CENTERED CARE

- Encourage the client to take measures to soften stools and promote bowel function (early ambulation, increased fluids, and high-fiber food sources).
- Administer stool softeners to prevent constipation.
- Enemas and suppositories are contraindicated for clients who have third- or fourth-degree perineal lacerations. Qs

Urinary system and bladder function

The urinary system can show evidence of the following.
- Urinary retention secondary to loss of bladder elasticity and tone and loss of bladder sensation resulting from trauma, medications, or anesthesia. A distended bladder as a result of urinary retention can cause uterine atony and displacement, decreasing the ability of the uterus to contract.
- Postpartum diuresis with increased urinary output begins within 12 hr of delivery.

DATA COLLECTION

Check the urinary system and bladder function.
- Determine the client's ability to void every 2 to 3 hr (perineal/urethral edema can cause pain and difficulty in voiding during the first 24 to 48 hr).
- Check bladder elimination pattern (client should be voiding every 2 to 3 hr). Excessive urine diuresis (more than 3,000 mL/day) is normal within the first 2 to 3 days after delivery.
- Check for evidence of a distended bladder.
  - Fundal height above the umbilicus or baseline level
  - Fundus displaced from the midline over to the side
  - Bladder bulges above the symphysis pubis
  - Excessive lochia
  - Tenderness over the bladder area
- Frequent voiding of less than 150 mL of urine is indicative of urinary retention with overflow.

PATIENT-CENTERED CARE

- Encourage the client to empty her bladder frequently (every 2 to 3 hr) to prevent possible displacement of the uterus and atony.
- Methods to induce voiding include assisting the client to the bathroom, running water in the sink or over the perineum, and providing privacy.
- Measure the first few voidings after delivery to determine bladder emptying.
- Encourage the client to increase oral fluid intake to replace fluids lost at delivery and to prevent or correct dehydration.
- Catheterize if necessary for bladder distention if the client is unable to void to ensure complete emptying of the bladder and allow uterine involution.

Musculoskeletal system

Physical changes of the musculoskeletal system involve a reversal of the musculoskeletal adaptations that occurred during pregnancy. By 6 to 8 weeks after birth:
- The joints return to their prepregnant state and are completely restabilized. The feet can remain permanently increased in size.
- Muscle tone begins to be restored throughout the body with the removal of progesterone's effect following delivery of the placenta. The rectus abdominis muscles of the abdomen and the pubococcygeus muscle tone are restored following placental expulsion and return to the prepregnant state about 6 weeks postpartum.

DATA COLLECTION

- Check the musculoskeletal system for changes.
- Check the abdominal wall for diastasis recti (separation of the rectus muscle) from 2 to 4 cm. It usually resolves within 6 weeks.

PATIENT-CENTERED CARE

- Reinforce teaching with the client on postpartum strengthening exercises.
  - Start with simple exercises.
  - Gradually progress to more strenuous exercises.
- Instruct clients who have had a cesarean birth to postpone strenuous exercise, abdominal exercise, heavy lifting, or excessive stair climbing until about 4 to 6 weeks following delivery, or as recommended by the provider.

CLIENT EDUCATION

- Do not perform housework requiring heavy lifting for at least 3 weeks. Do not lift anything heavier than the infant.
- Use good body mechanics and maintain proper posture.
- Avoid sitting for prolonged periods of time with legs crossed (to prevent thrombophlebitis).
- Do not drive for the first 2 weeks postpartum or while taking opioids for pain control.

Immune system

Review the status of the following.

Rubella: A client who has a titer of less than 1:8 will receive a subcutaneous injection of rubella vaccine or a measles, mumps, and rubella (MMR) vaccine during the postpartum period to protect a subsequent fetus from malformations. Caution the client to avoid getting pregnant for 28 days following the immunization due to the potential risk of birth defects in the fetus. Qs

Hepatitis B: Newborns born to infected mothers should receive the hepatitis B vaccine and hepatitis B immune globulin within 12 hr of birth.

Rh: All Rh-negative mothers who have newborns who are Rh-positive must receive IM Rho(D) immune globulin within 72 hr of the newborn being born to suppress antibody formation in the mother.
- Test the client who receives both the rubella vaccine and Rho(D) immune globulin after 3 months to determine whether immunity to rubella is evident. QEBP

Varicella: If the client has no immunity, the varicella vaccine is administered before discharge. Caution the client to avoid getting pregnant for 1 month following the immunization. A second dose of the vaccine is given at 4 to 8 weeks.

Tetanus–diphtheria–acellular pertussis vaccine: The vaccine is recommended for clients who have not previously received it. Administer prior to discharge or as soon as possible during the postpartum period.

Comfort level

DATA COLLECTION

- Check pain related to episiotomy, lacerations, incisions, afterpains, and sore nipples.
- Determine the location, type, and quality of the pain to guide nursing interventions and reinforce client education.

PATIENT-CENTERED CARE

The client should be discharged with an appointment date and time for a postpartum follow-up visit or a number to call and schedule an appointment.

- Following a vaginal delivery, the follow-up visit should take place in 4 to 6 weeks; following a cesarean birth, the visit should take place in 2 weeks.
- The date and time of the follow-up appointment should be written on the client's discharge paperwork and discussed in the discharge instructions.

CLIENT EDUCATION: Report the following indications of potential complications to the provider.

- Chills or fever greater than 38° C (100.4° F) for 2 or more days
- Change in vaginal discharge (increased amount, large clots, change to a previous lochia color, foul odor) Qs
- Episiotomy, laceration, or incisional pain, that is red, swollen, has foul smelling drainage, and not relieved with analgesics
- Pain or tenderness in the abdomen or pelvic area that is not relieved with analgesics
- Breasts with localized areas of pain, tenderness, heat, or swelling
- Nipples with cracks, redness, bruising, blisters, or fissures
- Calves with localized pain, tenderness, redness, and swelling
- A lower extremity with various areas of redness and warmth or coolness and paleness
- Burning, pain, frequency, or urgency upon urination
- Urine that is cloudy or contains blood
- Postpartum depression or feeling apathy toward the infant; inability to provide self-care or care for the infant; or feelings that she might hurt herself or her infant

1. A nurse is inspecting the perineal pad of a client who is 24 hr postpartum. The pad is saturated with approximately 12 cm of dark-red discharge. Which of the following blood loss estimations should the nurse report to the charge nurse and document in the client's medical record?

   A. Moderate

   B. Heavy

   C. Light

   D. Scant

2. A nurse is reinforcing discharge teaching with a postpartum client who had no immunity to varicella and received the varicella vaccine. Which of the following client statements indicates understanding of the teaching?

   A. "I will need to use contraception for 3 months before considering pregnancy."

   B. "I need a second vaccination at my postpartum visit."

   C. "I was given the vaccine because my baby is O-positive."

   D. "I will be tested in 3 months to see if I have developed immunity."

3. A nurse is reinforcing teaching with a client who is 1 week postpartum and breastfeeding. The client reports breast engorgement. Which of the following instructions should the nurse give to the client?

   A. "Apply cold compresses between feedings."

   B. "Take a warm shower right after feedings."

   C. "Apply breast milk to the nipples and allow them to air dry."

   D. "Use the various infant positions for feedings."

4. A nurse is reinforcing discharge instructions with a client who is 4 weeks postpartum. The nurse should instruct the client to contact her provider for which of the following findings?

   A. Scant, nonodorous white vaginal discharge

   B. Uterine cramping during breastfeeding

   C. Sore nipple with cracks and fissures

   D. Decreased response with sexual activity

5. A nurse is reinforcing discharge teaching with a postpartum client following a cesarean birth. The client reports leaking urine every time she sneezes or coughs. Which of the following interventions should the nurse suggest to the client?

   A. Sit-ups

   B. Pelvic tilt exercises

   C. Kegel exercises

   D. Abdominal crunches

PRACTICE Active Learning Scenario

A nurse on the postpartum unit is assisting the charge nurse prepare for a discussion with a group of clients about perineal care after delivery. What information should the nurse contribute for the discussion? Use the ATI Active Learning Template: Basic Concept to complete this item.

UNDERLYING PRINCIPLES: Describe three concepts that are the basis for perineal hygiene.

NURSING INTERVENTIONS

- Describe four actions the client should take to prevent infection.

- Describe four actions the nurse can take to promote client comfort.

Application Exercises Key

1. A. **CORRECT:** Moderate blood loss is greater than 10 cm. This is an expected finding 24 hr postpartum.

    B. Heavy blood loss is estimated as saturation of a perineal pad within 2 hr.

    C. Light blood loss is estimated as 2.5 to 10 cm of lochia on the perineal pad.

    D. Scant blood loss is estimated as less than 2.5 cm of lochia on the perineal pad.

    Ⓝ *NCLEX® Connection: Health Promotion and Maintenance, Ante/ Intra/Postpartum and Newborn Care*

2. A. A client is instructed to not get pregnant for 1 month following administration of varicella vaccine.

    B. **CORRECT:** A second varicella immunization is recommended at 4 to 8 weeks following delivery by clients who had no history of immunity.

    C. Rho(D) immune globulin is administered to a Rh-negative mother who has an Rh-positive newborn.

    D. A client requires testing for immunity at 3 months following administration of rubella vaccine and Rho(D) immune globulin.

    Ⓝ *NCLEX® Connection: Health Promotion and Maintenance, Health Promotion/Disease Prevention*

3. A. **CORRECT:** The nurse should instruct the client to apply cold compresses to the breasts after feedings to help with breast engorgement.

    B. Taking a warm shower prior to feedings, not immediately after, can assist with the letdown reflex and milk flow.

    C. Applying breast milk to the nipples and air drying is recommended for the client who has sore nipples, but it has no effect on breast engorgement.

    D. Using the various positions for feedings helps prevent nipple soreness but has no effect on breast engorgement.

    Ⓝ *NCLEX® Connection: Physiological Adaptation, Alterations in Body Systems*

4. A. Lochia alba, a white vaginal discharge, is an expected finding from the 11th day postpartum to approximately 6 weeks following birth.

    B. Oxytocin, which is released with breastfeeding, causes the uterus to contract and can cause discomfort.

    C. **CORRECT:** The nurse should instruct the client to contact the provider of sore nipples with cracks and fissures because this is an indication of mastitis, inflammation of the breast tissue.

    D. Physiological reactions to sexual activity can be slower and less intense for the first 3 months following birth.

    Ⓝ *NCLEX® Connection: Physiological Adaptation, Alterations in Body Systems*

5. A. Sit-ups should not be performed until after the postpartum follow-up appointment.

    B. Pelvic tilt exercises consist of the alternate arching and straightening of the back to strengthen the back muscles and relieve back discomfort.

    C. **CORRECT:** The nurse should suggest that the client perform Kegel exercises, which consist of the voluntary contraction and relaxation of the pubococcygeus muscle to strengthen the pelvic muscles. These exercises assist in decreasing postpartum urinary stress incontinence that occurs with sneezing and coughing.

    D. Abdominal crunches should not be performed until after the postpartum follow-up appointment.

    Ⓝ *NCLEX® Connection: Basic Care and Comfort, Elimination*

PRACTICE Answer

Using the ATI Active Learning Template: Basic Concept

UNDERLYING PRINCIPLES
- Promote stool softening.
- Promote comfort.

NURSING INTERVENTIONS
- Prevent infection.
  - Wash hands thoroughly before and after voiding.
  - Use a squeeze bottle filled with tap water warmed to 38° C (100.4°F) after each voiding to cleanse the perineal area.
  - Clean the perineal area from front to back.
  - Blot dry; do not wipe.
  - Sparingly use a topical application of antiseptic cream or spray 3 to 4 times daily.
  - Change perineal pad from front to back after voiding and defecating.

- Promote comfort.
  - Apply ice packs to the perineum for 24 to 48 hr.
  - Encourage sitz baths at least twice a day for 20 minutes.
  - Apply topical anesthetics to perineal area or witch hazel compresses to the rectal area 3 to 4 times daily.

Ⓝ *NCLEX® Connection: Health Promotion and Maintenance, Ante/Intra/Postpartum and Newborn Care*

UNIT 3   POSTPARTUM NURSING CARE

CHAPTER 13   *Complications of the Postpartum Period*

Postpartum Disorders

Postpartum disorders are unexpected events or occurrences that can happen during the postpartum period. It is important to have a thorough understanding of each disorder and implement evidence-based nursing interventions to achieve positive outcomes.

Postpartum disorders include superficial and deep-vein thrombosis, pulmonary embolus, postpartum hemorrhage, uterine atony, subinvolution of the uterus, inversion of the uterus, retained placenta, lacerations, and hematomas.

Deep-vein thrombosis

- Thrombophlebitis refers to a thrombus that is associated with inflammation.
- Thrombophlebitis of the lower extremities can be of superficial or deep veins, which are most often of the femoral, saphenous, or popliteal veins. The postpartum client is at risk for a deep-vein thrombosis (DVT) that can lead to a pulmonary embolism.

DATA COLLECTION

RISK FACTORS

- Pregnancy
- Cesarean birth (doubles the risk)
- Operative vaginal birth
- Pulmonary embolism or varicosities
- Immobility
- Obesity
- Smoking
- Multiparity
- Age greater than 35 years
- History of thromboembolism
- Diabetes mellitus

EXPECTED FINDINGS

Leg pain and tenderness

PHYSICAL FINDINGS
- Unilateral area of swelling, warmth, and redness
- Hardened vein over the thrombosis
- Calf tenderness

DIAGNOSTIC PROCEDURES

NONINVASIVE
- Doppler ultrasound scanning
- Computed tomography
- Magnetic resonance imaging

PATIENT-CENTERED CARE

NURSING CARE

Prevention of thrombophlebitis

- Measure the lower extremities for fitted elastic thromboembolic hose.
- Provide thigh-high antiembolism stockings for the client at high risk for venous insufficiency.
- Maintain sequential compression device until ambulation established.
- If bed rest is prolonged longer than 8 hr, perform active and passive range of motion to promote circulation in the legs if warranted.
- Initiate early and frequent ambulation postpartum.

CLIENT EDUCATION
- Follow instructions for measures to prevent DVT.
- Avoid prolonged periods of standing, sitting, or immobility.
- Elevate legs when sitting.
- Avoid crossing legs, which will reduce the circulation and exacerbate venous stasis.
- Maintain fluid intake of 2 to 3 L each day from food and beverage sources to prevent dehydration, which causes circulation to be sluggish.
- Stop smoking.

Management of thrombophlebitis

- Encourage rest.
- Facilitate bed rest and elevation of the extremity above the level of client's heart. (Avoid using a knee gatch or pillow under knees.)
- Administer intermittent or continuous warm moist compresses.
- Do **NOT** massage the affected limb to prevent thrombus from dislodging and becoming an embolus. Qs
- Measure and monitor the client's leg circumferences.
- Administer analgesics (nonsteroidal anti–inflammatory agents).
- Administer anticoagulants.

MEDICATIONS

Heparin

CLASSIFICATION: Anticoagulant

THERAPEUTIC INTENT: Given IV to prevent formation of other clots and to prevent enlargement of the existing clot.

NURSING ACTIONS
- Initially, heparin is administered by an RN via a continuous IV infusion for 3 to 5 days with doses adjusted according to coagulation studies. Protamine sulfate, the heparin antidote, should be readily available.
- Monitor aPTT (1.5 to 2.5 times the control level of 30 to 40 seconds).

CLIENT EDUCATION: Report bleeding from the gums or nose, increased vaginal bleeding, blood in the urine, and frequent bruising.

Warfarin

CLASSIFICATION: Anticoagulant

THERAPEUTIC INTENT: Used for treatment of clots. Administered orally and is continued by the client for approximately 3 months.

NURSING ACTIONS
- Phytonadione, the warfarin antidote, should be readily available for prolonged clotting times.
- Monitor PT (1.5 to 2.5 times the control level of 11 to 12.5 seconds) and INR of 2 to 3.

CLIENT EDUCATION
- Watch for bleeding from the gums or nose, increased vaginal bleeding, blood in the urine, and frequent bruising. Qs
- Use birth control to avoid pregnancy due to the teratogenic effects of warfarin. Oral contraceptives are contraindicated due to the increased risk for thrombosis.

CLIENT EDUCATION

PRECAUTIONS WHILE RECEIVING ANTICOAGULANTS QEBP
- Avoid taking aspirin or ibuprofen (increases bleeding tendencies).
- Use an electric razor for shaving.
- Avoid alcohol use (inhibits warfarin).
- Brush teeth gently using a soft toothbrush.
- Avoid rubbing or massaging legs.
- Avoid periods of prolonged sitting or crossing legs.

Pulmonary embolus

- An embolus occurs when fragments or an entire clot dislodges and moves into circulation.
- A pulmonary embolism is a complication of DVT that occurs if the embolus moves into the pulmonary artery or one of its branches and lodges in a lung, occluding the vessel and obstructing blood flow to the lungs.
- Acute pulmonary embolus is an emergent situation.

DATA COLLECTION

RISK FACTORS

Risk factors are the same as those for DVT.

EXPECTED FINDINGS
- Apprehension
- Pleuritic chest pain
- Dyspnea
- Tachypnea
- Hemoptysis
- Heart murmurs
- Peripheral edema
- Distended neck veins
- Elevated temperature
- Hypotension
- Hypoxia

DIAGNOSTIC AND THERAPEUTIC PROCEDURES
- Ventilation/perfusion lung scan
- Chest radiographic study
- Radioisotope lung scan
- Pulmonary angiogram
- Embolectomy to surgically remove the embolus

PATIENT-CENTERED CARE

NURSING CARE
- Place the client in a semi-Fowler's position with the head of the bed elevated to facilitate breathing.
- Administer oxygen by mask.

MEDICATIONS
- Medications prescribed include those for DVT.
- Thrombolytic therapy to break up blood clots may be prescribed by the provider and administered by an RN.

Postpartum hemorrhage

Postpartum hemorrhage is considered to occur if the client loses more than 500 mL of blood after a vaginal birth or more than 1,000 mL of blood after a cesarean birth. Two complications that can occur following postpartum hemorrhage are hypovolemic shock and anemia.

DATA COLLECTION

RISK FACTORS

- Uterine atony
- Overdistended uterus
- Previous history of uterine atony
- Prolonged or oxytocin-induced labor
- High parity
- Ruptured uterus
- Complications during pregnancy (placenta previa, abruptio placentae)
- Precipitous delivery
- Magnesium sulfate therapy during labor
- Lacerations and hematomas
- Inversion of uterus
- Subinvolution of the uterus
- Retained placental fragments
- Coagulopathies (DIC)

EXPECTED FINDINGS

Increase or change in lochia pattern (return to previous stage, large clots)

PHYSICAL FINDINGS
- Uterine atony (hypotonic or boggy)
- Blood clots larger than a quarter
- Perineal pad saturation in 15 min or less
- Constant oozing, trickling, or frank flow of bright red blood from the vagina
- Tachycardia and hypotension
- Skin pale, cool, and clammy with loss of turgor and pale mucous membranes
- Oliguria

LABORATORY TESTS

- Hgb and Hct
- Coagulation profile (PT)
- Blood type and crossmatch

PATIENT-CENTERED CARE

NURSING CARE

- Firmly massage the uterine fundus.
- Monitor vital signs.
- Monitor for source of bleeding.
  - Palpate fundus for height, firmness, and position. If uterus is boggy, massage fundus to increase muscle contraction.
  - Monitor lochia for color, quantity, and clots.
  - Observe for manifestations of bleeding from lacerations, episiotomy site, or hematomas.
- Palpate bladder for distention. Insert an indwelling urinary catheter to check kidney function and obtain an accurate measurement of urinary output.
- Maintain IV fluids to replace fluid volume loss with IV isotonic solutions (lactated Ringer's, 0.9% sodium chloride).
- Assist with administration of colloid volume expanders (such as albumin) and blood products (packed RBCs, fresh frozen plasma).
- Provide oxygen at 2 to 3 L/min per nasal cannula, and monitor oxygen saturation.
- Elevate the client's legs to 20° to 30° to increase venous return.

MEDICATIONS

Oxytocin

CLASSIFICATION: Uterine stimulant

THERAPEUTIC INTENT: Promote uterine contractions

NURSING ACTIONS
- Monitor uterine tone and vaginal bleeding.
- Monitor for adverse reaction of water intoxication (lightheadedness, nausea, vomiting, headache, malaise). This adverse effect can progress to cerebral edema with seizures, coma, and death.

Methylergonovine

CLASSIFICATION: Uterine stimulant

THERAPEUTIC INTENT: Control postpartum hemorrhage

NURSING ACTIONS
- Monitor uterine tone and vaginal bleeding. Do not administer to clients who have hypertension.
- Monitor for adverse reactions (hypertension, nausea, vomiting, headache).

Misoprostol

CLASSIFICATION: Uterine stimulant

THERAPEUTIC INTENT: Control postpartum hemorrhage.

NURSING ACTIONS: Monitor uterine tone and vaginal bleeding.

Carboprost tromethamine

CLASSIFICATION: Uterine stimulant

THERAPEUTIC INTENT: Control postpartum hemorrhage

NURSING ACTIONS
- Monitor uterine tone and vaginal bleeding.
- Monitor for adverse reactions (fever, chills, headache, nausea, vomiting, diarrhea).

CLIENT EDUCATION

- Limit physical activity to conserve strength.
- Increase iron and protein intake to promote the rebuilding of RBC volume.
- Take iron with vitamin C to enhance absorption.

Uterine atony

Uterine atony results from the inability of the uterine muscle to contract adequately after birth. This can lead to postpartum hemorrhage.

DATA COLLECTION

RISK FACTORS

- Retained placental fragments
- Prolonged labor
- Oxytocin induction or augmentation of labor
- Overdistention of the uterine muscle (multiparity, multiple gestations, polyhydramnios [hydramnios], macrosomic fetus)
- Precipitous labor
- Magnesium sulfate administration as a tocolytic
- Anesthesia and analgesia administration
- Trauma during labor and birth from operative delivery (forceps- or vacuum-assisted birth, cesarean birth)

EXPECTED FINDINGS

Increased vaginal bleeding

PHYSICAL FINDINGS
- Uterus that is larger than normal and boggy with possible lateral displacement on palpation
- Prolonged lochia discharge
- Irregular or excessive bleeding
- Tachycardia and hypotension
- Skin that is pale, cool, and clammy with loss of turgor and pale mucous membranes

DIAGNOSTIC PROCEDURES

- Bimanual compression or manual exploration of the uterine cavity for retained placental fragments by the provider
- Surgical management, such as hysterectomy

PATIENT-CENTERED CARE

NURSING CARE

- Ensure that the urinary bladder is empty.
- Monitor the following.
  - Fundal height, consistency, and location
  - Lochia for quantity, color, and consistency
- Perform fundal massage if indicated.
  - If the uterus becomes firm, continue monitoring.
  - If uterine atony persists, anticipate surgical intervention, such as a hysterectomy.
- Express clots that have accumulated in the uterus, but only after the uterus is firmly contracted. It is critical not to express clots prior to the uterus becoming firmly contracted because pushing on an uncontracted uterus can invert the uterus and result in extensive hemorrhage. Q EBP
- Monitor vital signs.
- Maintain IV fluids.
- Provide oxygen at 2 to 3 L/min per nasal cannula.

MEDICATIONS

As noted for postpartum hemorrhage

CLIENT EDUCATION

- Limit physical activity to conserve strength.
- Increase iron and protein intake to promote the rebuilding of RBC volume.

Subinvolution of the uterus

Subinvolution is when the uterus remains enlarged with continued lochia discharge and can result in postpartum hemorrhage.

DATA COLLECTION

RISK FACTORS

- Pelvic infection and endometritis
- Retained placental fragments not completely expelled from the uterus

EXPECTED FINDINGS

- Prolonged vaginal bleeding
- Irregular or excessive vaginal bleeding

PHYSICAL FINDINGS
- Uterus that is enlarged and higher than normal in the abdomen relative to the umbilicus
- Boggy uterus
- Prolonged lochia discharge with irregular or excessive bleeding

LABORATORY TESTS

Blood, intracervical, and intrauterine bacterial cultures to check for evidence of infection and endometritis

DIAGNOSTIC PROCEDURES

Dilation and curettage (D&C) is performed by the provider to remove retained placental fragments if indicated.

PATIENT-CENTERED CARE

NURSING CARE

- Monitor fundal position and consistency.
- Monitor lochia for color, amount, consistency, and odor.
- Monitor vital signs.
- Encourage the client to use activities that can enhance uterine involution. Q︎EBP
  - Breastfeeding
  - Early and frequent ambulation
  - Frequent voiding
- D&C can be necessary to remove retained placental fragments.

MEDICATIONS

Oxytocin, methylergonovine

CLASSIFICATION: Uterine stimulant

THERAPEUTIC INTENT: Promote uterine contractions and expel the retained fragments of placenta.

NURSING ACTIONS
- Monitor uterine tone and vaginal bleeding.
- Monitor for adverse reaction of water intoxication (lightheadedness, nausea, vomiting, headache, malaise), which can progress to cerebral edema with seizures, coma, and death.

Antibiotic therapy

Can be prescribed to prevent or treat infection

Inversion of the uterus

Inversion of the uterus is the turning inside out of the uterus. It can be partial or complete. Uterine inversion is an emergency situation that can result in postpartum hemorrhage and requires immediate intervention.

DATA COLLECTION

RISK FACTORS

- Retained placenta
- Uterine atony
- Vigorous fundal pressure
- Abnormally adherent placental tissue
- Fundal implantation of the placenta
- Excessive traction applied to the umbilical cord
- Short umbilical cord
- Prolonged labor

EXPECTED FINDINGS

Pain in lower abdomen

PHYSICAL FINDINGS
- Vaginal bleeding: hemorrhage
  - Complete inversion as evidenced by a large, red, rounded mass that protrudes 20 to 30 cm outside the introitus
  - Partial inversion as evidenced by the palpation of a smooth mass through the dilated cervix
- Dizziness
- Low blood pressure, increased pulse rate (shock)
- Pallor

DIAGNOSTIC PROCEDURES

Manual replacement of the uterus into the uterine cavity and repositioning of the uterus by the provider

PATIENT-CENTERED CARE

NURSING CARE

- Monitor for an inverted uterus.
  - Visualize the introitus.
  - Assist with a pelvic exam.
  - Maintain IV fluids.
  - Administer oxygen.
- Stop oxytocin if it is being administered at the time uterine inversion occurred.
- Anticipate surgery if nonsurgical interventions and management are unsuccessful.

MEDICATIONS

Terbutaline

CLASSIFICATION: Tocolytic

THERAPEUTIC INTENT: To relax the uterus prior to the provider's attempt at replacement of the uterus into the uterine cavity and uterus repositioning

NURSING ACTIONS
Following replacement of the uterus into the uterine cavity
- Closely observe the client's response to treatment.
- Monitor vital signs.
- Avoid aggressive fundal massage.
- Administer broad-spectrum antibiotics for infection prophylaxis.

CLIENT EDUCATION: A cesarean birth will be needed for subsequent pregnancies.

Retained placenta

The placenta or fragments of the placenta remain in the uterus and prevent the uterus from contracting, which can lead to uterine atony or subinvolution.

DATA COLLECTION

RISK FACTORS

- Partial separation of a normal placenta
- Entrapment of a partially or completely separated placenta by a constricting ring of the uterus
- Excessive traction on the umbilical cord prior to complete separation of the placenta
- Placental tissue that is abnormally adherent to the uterine wall
- Preterm birth between 20 and 24 weeks of gestation

EXPECTED FINDINGS

PHYSICAL FINDINGS
- Uterine atony, subinvolution, or inversion
- Excessive bleeding or blood clots larger than a quarter
- Return of lochia rubra once lochia has progressed to serosa or alba
- Malodorous lochia or vaginal discharge
- Elevated temperature

LABORATORY TESTS

Hgb and Hct

DIAGNOSTIC PROCEDURES

- Manual separation and removal of the placenta is done by the provider.
- D&C performed by the provider if oxytocics are ineffective in expelling the placental fragments.

PATIENT-CENTERED CARE

NURSING CARE

- Monitor the uterus for fundal height, consistency, and position.
- Monitor lochia for color, amount, consistency, and odor.
- Monitor vital signs.
- Maintain IV fluids.
- Provide oxygen at 2 to 3 L/min per nasal cannula.
- Anticipate surgical interventions (D&C, hysterectomy) if postpartum bleeding continues.

MEDICATIONS

Oxytocin

To expel retained fragments of the placenta

CLASSIFICATION: Uterine stimulant

THERAPEUTIC INTENT: Promote uterine contractions and expel the retained fragments of placenta

Terbutaline

CLASSIFICATION: Tocolytic

THERAPEUTIC INTENT: Relax the uterus prior to D&C if placental expulsion with oxytocics is unsuccessful

CLIENT EDUCATION

- Limit physical activity to conserve strength.
- Increase iron and protein intake to promote the rebuilding of RBC volume.

Lacerations and hematomas

- Lacerations that occur during labor and birth consist of the tearing of soft tissues in the birth canal and adjacent structures including the cervical, vaginal, vulvar, perineal, and rectal areas.
- An episiotomy can extend and become a third- or fourth-degree laceration.
- A hematoma is a collection of 250 to 500 mL of clotted blood within tissues that can appear as a bulging bluish mass. Hematomas can occur in the pelvic region or higher in the vagina or broad ligament.
- Pain, rather than noticeable bleeding, is the distinguishable manifestation of hematomas.
- The client is at risk for hemorrhage or infection due to a laceration or hematoma.

DATA COLLECTION

RISK FACTORS

- Operative vaginal birth (forceps- or vacuum-assisted)
- Precipitous birth
- Cephalopelvic disproportion
- Size (macrosomic infant) and abnormal presentation or position of the fetus
- Prolonged pressure of the fetal head on the vaginal mucosa
- Previous scarring of the birth canal from infection, injury, or operation
- Clients who are nulliparous are at a greater risk for injury due to firmer and less resistant tissue.
- Clients who have light skin, especially those with reddish hair, have less distensible tissue than clients who have dark skin.

EXPECTED FINDINGS

Laceration
- Sensation of oozing or trickling of blood
- Excessive rubra lochia (with or without clots)

Hematoma
- Pain
- Pressure sensation in rectum (urge to defecate) or vagina
- Difficulty voiding

PHYSICAL FINDINGS
- **Laceration**
  - Vaginal bleeding even though the uterus is firm and contracted
  - Continuous slow trickle of bright red blood from vagina, laceration, episiotomy
- **Hematoma:** Bulging, bluish mass or area of red-purple discoloration on vulva, perineum, or rectum

PATIENT-CENTERED CARE

NURSING CARE

- Monitor pain.
- Visually or manually inspect the vulva, perineum, and rectum for lacerations and hematomas.
- Monitor an episiotomy for extension into a third- or fourth-degree laceration.
- Evaluate lochia.
- Continue to monitor vital signs and hemodynamic status.
- Attempt to identify the source of the bleeding.
- Assist the provider with repair procedures.
- Use ice packs to treat small hematomas.
- Administer pain medication.
- Encourage sitz baths and frequent perineal hygiene.

THERAPEUTIC PROCEDURES

- Repair and suturing of the episiotomy or lacerations is done by the provider.
- Ligation of the bleeding vessel or surgical incision for evacuation of the clotted blood from the hematoma is done by the provider.

Postpartum Infections

Postpartum infections can occur up to 28 days following childbirth or spontaneous or induced abortion. Fever of 38° C (100.4° F) or higher for 2 consecutive days during the first 10 days of the postpartum period indicates postpartum infection and requires further investigation.

Uterine infection, wound infection, mastitis, and urinary tract infection are examples of postpartum infections. Early identification and prompt treatment are necessary to promote positive outcomes.

Infections (endometritis, mastitis, wound infections)

Uterine infection is also referred to as **endometritis**.
- Endometritis is an infection of the uterine lining or endometrium. It is the most frequently occurring puerperal infection.
- Endometritis usually begins on the second to fifth postpartum day, generally starting as a localized infection at the placental attachment site and spreading to include the entire uterine endometrium.

Wound infection sites include cesarean incisions, episiotomies, lacerations, and any trauma wounds in the birth canal following labor and birth.

Mastitis is an infection of the breast involving the interlobular connective tissue and is usually unilateral. Mastitis can progress to an abscess if untreated.
- It occurs most commonly in mothers breastfeeding for the first time and well after the establishment of milk flow (usually 6 weeks after delivery).
- *Staphylococcus aureus* is usually the infecting organism.

DATA COLLECTION

RISK FACTORS

The immediate postpartum period following birth is a time of increased risk for all clients for micro-organisms entering the reproductive tract and migrating into the blood and other parts of the body, which can result in life-threatening septicemia.
- Urinary tract infection, mastitis, pneumonia, or history of previous venous thrombus
- History of diabetes mellitus, immunosuppression, anemia, or malnutrition
- History of alcohol or other substance use disorder
- Cervical dilation that provides the uterus with exposure to the external environment through the vagina

- Well-supplied exposed blood vessels
- Wounds from lacerations, incisions, or hematomas
- Alkalinity of amniotic fluid, blood, and lochia during pregnancy and the early postpartum period, decreasing the acidity of the vaginal secretions
- Cesarean birth
- Prolonged rupture of membranes
- Retained placental fragments and manual extraction of the placenta
- Chorioamnionitis
- Internal fetal/uterine pressure monitoring
- Multiple vaginal examinations after rupture of membranes
- Prolonged labor
- Postpartum hemorrhage
- Operative vaginal birth
- Epidural analgesia/anesthesia
- Hematomas
- Episiotomy or lacerations

Mastitis

- Milk stasis from a blocked duct
- Nipple trauma and cracked or fissured nipples
- Poor breastfeeding technique with improper latching of the infant onto the breast, which can lead to sore and cracked nipples
- Decrease in breastfeeding frequency due to supplementation with bottle feeding
- Poor hygiene and inadequate handwashing when handling perineal pads and touching the breasts

EXPECTED FINDINGS

Puerperal infections
- Flulike manifestations, such as body aches, chills, fever, and malaise
- Anorexia and nausea

Endometritis
- Pelvic pain
- Chills
- Fatigue
- Loss of appetite

Mastitis
- Painful or tender localized hard mass and reddened area, usually on one breast
- Chills
- Fatigue

PHYSICAL FINDINGS
- **Puerperal infections**
  - Temperature of at least 38° C (100.4° F) for 2 or more consecutive days
  - Tachycardia
- **Endometritis**
  - Uterine tenderness and enlargement
  - Dark, profuse lochia
  - Lochia that is either malodorous or purulent
  - Temperature greater than 38° C (100.4° F), typically on the third to fourth postpartum day
  - Tachycardia

- **Wound infection**
  - Wound warmth, erythema, tenderness, pain, edema, and seropurulent drainage
  - Wound dehiscence (separation of wound or incision edges) or evisceration (protrusion of internal contents through the separated wound edges)
  - Temperature greater than 38° C (100.4° F) for 2 or more consecutive days
- **Mastitis:** Axillary adenopathy in the affected side (enlarged tender axillary lymph nodes) with an area of inflammation that can be red, swollen, warm, and tender

LABORATORY TESTS

- Blood, intracervical, or intrauterine bacterial cultures to reveal the offending organism
- WBC count: leukocytosis
- RBC sedimentation rate: distinctly increased
- RBC count: anemia

PATIENT-CENTERED CARE

NURSING CARE

- Obtain frequent vital signs.
- Monitor pain.
- Monitor fundal height, position, and consistency.
- Observe lochia for color, quantity, and consistency.
- Inspect incisions, episiotomy, and lacerations.
- Inspect breasts.

Puerperal infections

- Use aseptic technique for sterile procedures; perform proper hand hygiene; and don gloves for labor, birth, and postpartum care.
- Reinforce client education about preventative measures to include thorough handwashing and good perineal hygiene.
- Maintain IV access.
- Assist with administration of IV broad-spectrum antibiotic therapy (penicillins or cephalosporins).
- Provide comfort measures (warm blankets, cool compresses) depending on findings.
- Reinforce teaching with the client about manifestations of worsening conditions to report and the importance of adherence to the treatment plan with the completion of a full course of antibiotics.
- Encourage a diet high in protein to promote tissue healing.

Endometritis

- Collect vaginal and blood cultures.
- Assist with administration of IV antibiotics.
- Administer analgesics.
- Reinforce teaching with the client about hand hygiene.
- Encourage the client to maintain interaction with the infant to facilitate bonding.

Wound infection

- Perform wound care.
- Administer IV antibiotics.
- Provide or encourage comfort measures (sitz baths, perineal care, warm or cold compresses).
- Reinforce teaching with the client about good hand hygiene techniques (removing perineal pads from front to back, performing thorough hand hygiene prior to and after perineal care).

Mastitis

- Reinforce teaching with the client about proper infant positioning and latching-on techniques, including both the nipple and the areola. The client should release the infant's grasp on the nipple prior to removing the infant from the breast. Q EBP
- Encourage rest, analgesics, and fluid intake of at least 3,000 mL per day.
- Administer antibiotics.
- Reinforce client education regarding breast hygiene to prevent and manage mastitis.

CLIENT EDUCATION

- Thoroughly wash hands prior to breastfeeding.
- Maintain cleanliness of breasts with frequent changes of breast pads.
- Allow nipples to air-dry.
- Completely empty breasts with each feeding to prevent milk stasis, which provides a medium for bacterial growth.
- Use ice packs or warm packs on affected breasts for discomfort.
- Continue breastfeeding frequently (at least every 2 to 4 hr), especially on the affected side.
- Manually express breast milk or use a breast pump if breastfeeding is too painful.
- Begin breastfeeding from the unaffected breast first to initiate the letdown reflex in the affected breast that is distended or tender.
- Wear a well-fitting bra for support.
- Report redness and fever.
- Complete the entire course of antibiotics as prescribed.

MEDICATIONS

For endometritis

Clindamycin, cephalosporins, penicillins, gentamicin

CLASSIFICATION: Antibiotic

THERAPEUTIC INTENT: Treatment of bacterial infections

CLIENT EDUCATION

- Take all the medication as prescribed.
- Notify the provider of the development of watery, bloody diarrhea.
- Notify the provider if breastfeeding.

THERAPEUTIC PROCEDURES

The provider might need to open and drain the wound or perform wound debridement if indicated.

Urinary tract infection

- Urinary tract infections (UTIs) are a common postpartum infection secondary to bladder trauma incurred during the delivery or a break in aseptic technique during bladder catheterization.
- A potential complication of a UTI is the progression to pyelonephritis with permanent kidney damage leading to chronic kidney disease.

DATA COLLECTION

RISK FACTORS

- Postpartal hypotonic bladder or urethra (urinary stasis and retention)
- Epidural anesthesia
- Urinary bladder catheterization
- Frequent pelvic examinations
- Genital tract injuries
- History of UTIs
- Cesarean birth

EXPECTED FINDINGS

- Reports of urgency, frequency, dysuria, and pelvic area discomfort
- Fever
- Chills
- Malaise

PHYSICAL FINDINGS

- Change in vital signs
- Elevated temperature
- Urine (cloudy, blood-tinged, malodorous, sediment visible)
- Urinary retention
- Pain in the suprapubic area
- Pain at the costovertebral angle (pyelonephritis)

DIAGNOSTIC PROCEDURES

Urinalysis for WBCs, RBCs, protein, bacteria

PATIENT-CENTERED CARE

NURSING CARE

- Obtain a random or clean-catch urine sample.
- Administer antibiotics. Acetaminophen reduces discomfort and pain associated with a urinary tract infection.
- Reinforce proper perineal hygiene, such as wiping from front to back.

CLIENT EDUCATION

- Increase fluid intake to 3,000 mL/day to dilute the bacteria and flush bladder.
- Complete the entire course of antibiotics as prescribed.
- Drink cranberry and prune juice to promote urine acidification, which inhibits bacterial multiplication. Q EBP

Postpartum Blues, Depression, and Psychosis

Postpartum blues can occur during the first few days after birth and generally continues for up to 10 days. Postpartum blues resolves without treatment.

Postpartum depression occurs within 12 months of delivery and is characterized by persistent feelings of sadness and intense mood swings. It usually does not resolve without treatment.

Postpartum psychosis develops within the first 2 to 3 weeks of the postpartum period. Clients who have a history of bipolar disorder are at increased risk. Manifestations are severe (confusion, disorientation, hallucinations, delusions, obsessive behaviors, paranoia). The client might attempt to harm herself or infant. Postpartum psychosis is an emergent situation that requires acute psychiatric treatment.

DATA COLLECTION

RISK FACTORS

- Hormonal changes with a rapid decline in estrogen and progesterone levels
- Postpartum physical discomfort or pain
- Individual socioeconomic factors
- Decreased social support system
- Anxiety about assuming new role as a mother
- Unplanned or unwanted pregnancy
- History of previous depressive disorder
- Low self-esteem
- History of intimate partner violence

EXPECTED FINDINGS

Postpartum blues

- Feelings of sadness
- Lack of appetite
- Sleep pattern disturbances
- Feeling of inadequacies
- Crying easily for no apparent reason
- Restlessness, insomnia, fatigue
- Headache
- Anxiety, anger, sadness

Postpartum depression

- Feelings of guilt and inadequacies
- Irritability
- Anxiety
- Fatigue persisting beyond a reasonable amount of time
- Feeling of loss
- Lack of appetite
- Persistent feelings of sadness
- Intense mood swings
- Sleep pattern disturbances

PHYSICAL FINDINGS
- Crying
- Weight loss
- Flat affect
- Irritability
- Rejection of the infant
- Severe anxiety and panic attack

Postpartum psychosis

- Pronounced sadness
- Disorientation
- Confusion
- Paranoia

PHYSICAL FINDINGS: Behaviors indicating hallucinations or delusional thoughts of self-harm or harming the infant

PATIENT-CENTERED CARE

NURSING CARE

- Monitor interactions between the client and infant. Encourage bonding activities.
- Monitor the client's mood and affect.
- Reinforce that feeling down in the postpartum period is expected and self-limiting. Encourage the client to notify the provider if the condition persists.
- Encourage the client to communicate feelings, validate and address personal conflicts, and reinforce personal power and autonomy.
- Reinforce the importance of compliance with any prescribed medication regimen.
- Contact a community resource to schedule a follow-up visit after discharge for clients who are at high risk for postpartum depression.
- Ask the client if she has thoughts of self-harm, suicide, or harming the infant. Provide for the safety of the infant and client as the priority of care. **Qs**

MEDICATIONS

Antidepressants may be prescribed for clients who have postpartum depression.

Antipsychotics and **mood stabilizers** may be prescribed for clients who have postpartum psychosis.

NURSING ACTIONS

CARE AFTER DISCHARGE

- Advise the client to get plenty of rest and to nap when the newborn sleeps.
- Reinforce the importance of the client taking time out for herself.
- Schedule a follow-up visit prior to the routine postpartum visit for clients who are at risk for developing postpartum depression.
- Provide information about community resources such as La Leche League or community mental health centers.
- Encourage the client to seek counseling. Make referrals to social agencies as indicated.

Application Exercises

1. A nurse on a postpartum unit is contributing to the plan of care for a client who has thrombophlebitis. Which of the following interventions should the nurse recommend?

   A. Apply cold compresses to the affected extremity.

   B. Massage the affected extremity.

   C. Allow the client to ambulate.

   D. Measure leg circumferences.

2. A nurse is reinforcing teaching with a client who is breastfeeding and has mastitis. Which of the following statements should the nurse make?

   A. "Limit the amount of time the infant nurses on each breast."

   B. "Nurse the infant only on the unaffected breast until resolved."

   C. "Completely empty each breast at each feeding or use a pump."

   D. "Wear a tight-fitting bra until lactation has ceased."

3. A nurse is discussing risks factors for urinary tract infections with a newly licensed nurse. Which of the following risk factors should the nurse include? (Select all that apply).

   A. Epidural anesthesia

   B. Urinary bladder catheterization

   C. Frequent pelvic examinations

   D. History of UTIs

   E. Vaginal birth

4. A nurse is collecting data from a postpartum client who is exhibiting tearfulness, insomnia, lack of appetite, and a feeling of sadness. The nurse should identify these findings as an indication of which of the following conditions?

   A. Postpartum fatigue

   B. Postpartum psychosis

   C. Postpartum endometritis

   D. Postpartum blues

5. A nurse is caring for a client who has postpartum psychosis. Which of the following actions is the nurse's priority?

   A. Reinforce the need to take antipsychotics as prescribed.

   B. Ask the client if she has thoughts of harming herself or her infant.

   C. Monitor the infant for indications of failure to thrive.

   D. Review the client's medical record for a history of bipolar disorder.

Application Exercises Key

1. A. The nurse should plan to apply warm compresses to the affected extremity.

   B. The nurse should not massage the affected extremity. This action can result in dislodgement of the clot.

   C. The client should be encouraged to rest with the affected extremity elevated.

   D. **CORRECT:** The nurse should measure the circumference of the leg to monitor for changes in the client's condition.

   Ⓝ *NCLEX® Connection: Physiological Adaptation, Alterations in Body Systems*

2. A. Frequent, on-demand breastfeeding should be encouraged to promote milk flow.

   B. The client should be instructed to continue breastfeeding, especially on the affected side.

   C. **CORRECT:** Instruct the client to completely empty each breast at each feeding to prevent milk stasis, which provides a medium for bacterial growth.

   D. The client should wear a well-fitting bra, not one that is too tight or a binder.

   Ⓝ *NCLEX® Connection: Health Promotion and Maintenance, Ante/Intra/Postpartum and Newborn Care*

3. A. **CORRECT:** Epidural anesthesia is a risk factor for a UTI.

   B. **CORRECT:** Urinary bladder catheterization is a risk factor for a UTI.

   C. **CORRECT:** A history of frequent pelvic examinations is a risk factor for a UTI.

   D. **CORRECT:** A history of UTIs is a risk factor for developing UTIs.

   B. Cesarean birth places a client at risk for development of a UTI.

   Ⓝ *NCLEX® Connection: Health Promotion and Maintenance, Health Promotion/Disease Prevention*

4. A. Postpartum fatigue results from the work of labor. It is usually self-limiting.

   B. The client who has postpartum psychosis will exhibit pronounced feelings of sadness, confusion, disorientation, hallucinations, delusions, and paranoia, and might attempt to harm herself or her infant.

   C. The client who has postpartum endometritis will exhibit fever, uterine tenderness, and foul-smelling vaginal discharge.

   D. **CORRECT:** Postpartum blues are characterized by tearfulness, insomnia, lack of appetite, and feelings of sadness or inadequacies.

   Ⓝ *NCLEX® Connection: Health Promotion and Maintenance, Developmental Stages and Transitions*

5. A. The nurse should reinforce the need to take antipsychotics as prescribed to manage the manifestations of postpartum psychosis. However, action is the priority.

   B. **CORRECT:** The greatest risk to the client and infant is self-harm or harm directed toward the infant.

   C. The nurse should monitor the infant for indications of failure to thrive as the client who has postpartum psychosis might be unable to provide care for the infant. However, action is the priority.

   D. The nurse should review the client's medical record for a history of bipolar disorder as this is associated with an increased risk for postpartum psychosis. However, action is the priority.

   Ⓝ *NCLEX® Connection: Health Promotion and Maintenance, Developmental Stages and Transitions*

PRACTICE Answer

Using the ATI Active Learning Template: System Disorder

ALTERATION IN HEALTH (DIAGNOSIS):
DVT refers to a thrombus that is associated with inflammation. It can occur in a superficial or deep vein (femoral, saphenous, popliteal).

RISK FACTORS
• Pregnancy
• Immobility
• Obesity
• Smoking
• Cesarean birth
• Multiparity
• Age greater than 35 years
• History of previous thromboembolism
• Diabetes mellitus

CLIENT EDUCATION
• Wear antiembolic stockings until ambulation established.
• Perform active range of motion when on bed rest for longer than 8 hr.
• Initiate early and frequent postpartum ambulation.
• Avoid prolonged periods of standing, sitting, or immobility.
• Elevate the legs when sitting.
• Avoid crossing legs.
• Maintain 2 to 3 L of daily fluid intake from food and beverage sources.
• Stop smoking.

MEDICATIONS
• Heparin: aPTT
• Warfarin: PT and INR

Ⓝ *NCLEX® Connection: Physiological Adaptation, Alterations in Body Systems*

NCLEX® Connections

When reviewing the following chapters, keep in mind the relevant topics and tasks of the NCLEX outline, in particular:

Safe and Effective Care Environment

HOME SAFETY: Provide the client with information on home safety.

SECURITY PLAN: Initiate and participate in security alert (infant abduction, flight risk).

Health Promotion and Maintenance

AGING PROCESS: Provide care that meets the needs of the newborn less than 1 month old through the infant or toddler client through 2 years.

ANTE/INTRA/POSTPARTUM AND NEWBORN CARE
Contribute to the newborn plan of care.

Reinforce client teaching on infant care skills (feeding, bathing, positioning).

DATA COLLECTION TECHNIQUES
Collect data for health history (client medical history, family medical history).

Collect baseline physical data (skin integrity, height and weight).

DEVELOPMENTAL STAGES AND TRANSITIONS
Identify and report client deviations from expected growth and development.

Assist client with expected life transition (attachment to newborn, parenting, retirement).

Pharmacological Therapies

EXPECTED ACTIONS/OUTCOMES
Apply knowledge of pathophysiology when addressing the client's pharmacological agents.

Evaluate the client's response to medication (adverse reactions, interactions, therapeutic effects).

Reduction of Risk Potential

POTENTIAL FOR COMPLICATIONS OF DIAGNOSTIC TESTS/TREATMENTS/PROCEDURES: Implement measures to prevent complication of client condition or procedure (circulatory complication, seizure, aspiration, potential neurological disorder).

Physiological Adaptation

ALTERATIONS IN BODY SYSTEMS

Identify signs and symptoms of an infection (temperature changes, swelling, redness, mental confusion, foul smelling urine).

Provide care for a client experiencing complications of pregnancy/labor and/or delivery (eclampsia, precipitous labor, hemorrhage).

FLUID AND ELECTROLYTE IMBALANCES: Identify signs and symptoms of client fluid and/or electrolyte imbalances.

CHAPTER 14

Newborn Data Collection

Understanding the physiologic and behavioral adjustment to being outside the uterus is imperative for providing newborn nursing care. Key responsibilities include assisting with the physical examination of the newborn, obtaining vital signs and measurements, recognizing classifications of the newborn by gestational age and weight, assisting with or observing diagnostic and therapeutic procedures, and recognizing complications.

PHYSIOLOGIC RESPONSE OF NEWBORN TO BIRTH

- Adjustments to extrauterine life occur as a newborn's respiratory and circulatory systems are required to rapidly adjust to life outside of the uterus.
- The establishment of respiratory function with the cutting of the umbilical cord is the most critical extrauterine adjustment as air inflates the lungs with the first breath.
- Circulatory changes after birth occur with the expulsion of the placenta and the cutting of the umbilical cord as a newborn begins breathing independently. The three shunts (ductus arteriosus, ductus venosus, foramen ovale) functionally close during a newborn's transition to extrauterine life with the flow of oxygenated blood in the lungs and readjustment of atrial blood pressure in the heart.

DATA COLLECTION OF NEWBORN FOLLOWING BIRTH

EQUIPMENT FOR DATA COLLECTION

Bulb syringe: Used for removing excess mucus from the mouth and nose.

Stethoscope with a pediatric head: Used to evaluate heart rate, breath sounds, and bowel sounds.

Axillary thermometer: Used to monitor temperature and prevent hypothermia. Rectal temperatures are avoided because they can injure the newborn's delicate rectal mucosa. An initial rectal temperature can be obtained to evaluate for anal abnormalities.

Blood pressure cuff 2.5 cm wide: Palpation or electronic method. Blood pressure can be done in all four extremities if evaluating the newborn for cardiac problems.

Scale with protective cover in place: Scale should be at 0; weight should include pounds, ounces, kilograms, and grams.

Tape measure in centimeters: Measure from crown to heel of foot for length. Measure head circumference at greatest diameter (occipital to frontal). Measure chest circumference beginning at the nipple line, and abdominal circumference above the umbilicus.

Clean gloves: Worn for all physical examinations until discharge.

BASELINE PHYSICAL DATA OF NEWBORN

External observations: Skin color, peeling, birthmarks, foot creases, breast tissue, nasal patency, and meconium staining (can indicate fetal hypoxia)

Chest: Point of maximal impulse location; ease of breathing; auscultation for heart rate and quality of tones; and respirations for crackles, wheezes, and equality of bilateral breath sounds

Abdomen: Rounded abdomen and umbilical cord with one vein and two arteries

Neurologic: Muscle tone and reflex reaction (Moro reflex); palpation for the presence and size of fontanels and sutures; palpation of fontanels for fullness or bulge

Other observations: Inspection for gross structural malformations

EXPECTED REFERENCE RANGES
- **Weight:** 2,500 to 4,000 g (5.51 to 8.81 lb)
- **Length:** 45 to 55 cm (17.7 to 21.6 in)
- **Head circumference:** 32 to 36.8 cm (12.6 to 14.5 in)
- **Chest circumference:** 30 to 33 cm (11.8 to 12.9 in)

CLASSIFICATION: Following data collection, classification of the newborn by gestational age and birth weight is determined.
- **Appropriate for gestational age (AGA):** Weight is between the 10th and 90th percentile.
- **Small for gestational age (SGA):** Weight is less than the 10th percentile.
- **Large for gestational age (LGA):** Weight is greater than the 90th percentile.
- **Low birth weight (LBW):** Weight is 2,500 g or less at birth.
- **Intrauterine growth restriction (IUGR):** Growth rate does not meet expected norms.
- **Term:** Birth between the beginning of week 37 and prior to the end of 42 weeks of gestation
- **Preterm or premature:** Born prior to the completion of 37 weeks of gestation
- **Postterm (postdate):** Born after the completion of 42 weeks of gestation
- **Postmature:** Born after the completion of 42 weeks of gestation with evidence of placental insufficiency

VITAL SIGNS

Vital signs are checked in the following sequence: respirations, heart rate, temperature. Blood pressure is not routinely measured unless there is a risk of cardiac problems. Newborns who have an irregular, very slow, or very fast heart rate should have a blood pressure measurement. The nurse observes the respiratory rate first before the newborn becomes active or agitated by use of the stethoscope, thermometer, or blood pressure cuff.

Respiratory rate varies from 30 to 60 breaths/min with short periods of apnea (less than 15 seconds) occurring most frequently during the rapid eye movement sleep cycle. Periods of apnea lasting longer than 15 seconds should be reported. Crackles and wheezing are manifestations of fluid or infection in the lungs. Grunting and nasal flaring are clinical findings of respiratory distress.

Expected heart rate ranges from 110 to 160/min with brief fluctuations above and below this range depending on activity level (crying, sleeping). Apical pulse rate is counted for 1 full minute, preferably when the newborn is sleeping. The pediatric stethoscope head is placed on the fourth or fifth intercostal space at the left midclavicular line over the apex of the newborn's heart. Heart murmurs are documented and reported.

Blood pressure should be 60 to 80 mm Hg systolic and 40 to 50 mm Hg diastolic.

Expected temperature range is 36.5° C to 37.5° C (97.7° F to 99.5° F) axillary. The newborn is at risk for hypothermia and hyperthermia until thermoregulation (ability to produce heat and maintain expected body temperature) stabilizes. If the newborn becomes chilled (cold stress), oxygen demands can increase and acidosis can occur.

14.1 Mongolian spots

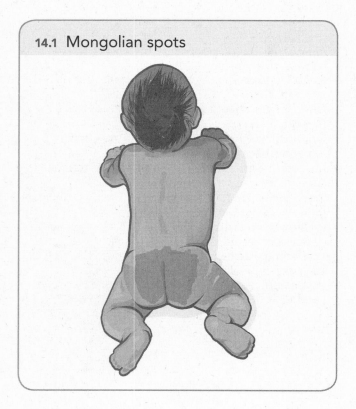

A more extensive physical exam is performed on the neonate within 24 hr of birth. Vital signs are obtained. A head-to-toe physical exam is performed. Neurological and behavioral evaluations are completed by eliciting reflexes and observing responses. Laboratory data is monitored.

PHYSICAL EXAM FROM HEAD TO TOE

Posture

- Lying in a curled-up position with arms and legs in moderate flexion
- Resistant to extension of extremities

Skin

- Skin color should be pink or acrocyanotic with no jaundice present on the first day. Secondary to increased bilirubin, jaundice can appear on the third day of life but then decrease spontaneously.
- Skin turgor should be present, showing that the newborn is well hydrated. The skin should spring back immediately when pinched.
- Texture should be dry, soft, and smooth, showing good hydration. Cracks in hands and feet can be present. In term newborns, desquamation (peeling) occurs a few days after birth.
- Vernix caseosa (protective, thick, cheesy covering) amounts vary, with more present in creases and skin folds.
- Lanugo (fine downy hair) varies regarding the amount present. It is usually found on the pinnae of ears, forehead, and shoulders.

EXPECTED DEVIATIONS
- **Milia** (small raised white spots on the nose, chin, and forehead) can be present. These spots disappear spontaneously without treatment (parents should not squeeze the spots).
- **Mongolian spots** (bluish purple spots of pigmentation) are commonly noted on the shoulders, back, and buttocks. These spots are frequently present on newborns of African American, Asian, or Native American origin. Be sure the parents are aware of Mongolian spots, and document location and presence. **(14.1)**
- **Telangiectatic nevi** (stork bites) are flat pink or red marks that easily blanch and are found on the back of the neck, nose, upper eyelids, and middle of the forehead. They usually fade by the second year of life. **(14.2)**
- **Nevus flammeus** (port wine stain) is a capillary angioma below the surface of the skin that is purple or red, varies in size and shape, is commonly seen on the face, and does not blanch or disappear.
- **Erythema toxicum** (erythema neonatorum) is a pink rash that appears suddenly anywhere on the body of a term newborn during the first 3 weeks. This is frequently referred to as newborn rash. No treatment is required.

Head

- Head circumference should be 2 to 3 cm larger than chest circumference. Head circumference greater than or equal to 4 cm larger than the chest circumference can be an indication of **hydrocephalus** (excessive cerebral fluid within the brain cavity surrounding the brain). Head circumference less than or equal to 32 cm can be an indication of **microcephaly** (abnormally small head).
- Anterior fontanel should be palpated and approximately 5 cm on average and diamond-shaped. Posterior fontanel is smaller and triangle-shaped. Fontanels should be soft and flat. Fontanels can bulge when the newborn cries, coughs, or vomits, and are flat when the newborn is quiet. Bulging fontanels can indicate increased intracranial pressure, infection, or hemorrhage. Depressed fontanels can indicate dehydration.
- Sutures should be palpable, separated, and can be overlapping (molding), an expected occurrence resulting from head compression during labor.
- **Caput succedaneum** (localized swelling of the soft tissues of the scalp caused by pressure on the head during labor) is an expected finding that can be palpated as a soft edematous mass and can cross over the suture line. Caput succedaneum usually resolves in 3 to 4 days and does not require treatment. **(14.3)**
- **Cephalohematoma** is a collection of blood between the periosteum and the skull bone that it covers. It does not cross the suture line. It results from trauma during birth such as pressure of the fetal head against the maternal pelvis in a prolonged difficult labor or forceps delivery. It appears in the first 1 to 2 days after birth and resolves in 2 to 3 weeks. **(14.4)**

Eyes

- Observe eyes for symmetry in size and shape.
- Each eye and the space between the eyes should equal one-third the distance from the inner to the outer canthus of both eyes to rule out chromosomal abnormalities, such as Down syndrome.
- Eyes are usually blue or gray following birth.
- Lacrimal glands are immature, with minimal or no tears.
- Subconjunctival hemorrhages can result from pressure during birth.
- Pupillary and red reflex are present.
- Eyeball movement will demonstrate random, jerky movements.

Ears

- When examining the placement of ears, draw an imaginary line through the inner to the outer canthus of the newborn's eye. The eye should be even with the upper tip of the pinna of the newborn's ear. Ears that are low-set can indicate a chromosomal abnormality, intellectual impairment, or kidney disease.
- Cartilage should be firm and well formed. Lack of cartilage indicates prematurity.
- The newborn should respond to voices and other sounds.
- Inspect ears for skin tags.

Nose

- The nose should be midline, flat, and broad with lack of a bridge.
- Some mucus should be present, but with no drainage.
- Newborns are obligate nose breathers and do not develop the response of opening the mouth with a nasal obstruction until 3 weeks after birth. Therefore, a nasal blockage can result in flaring of the nares, cyanosis, or asphyxia.
- Newborns sneeze to clear nasal passages.

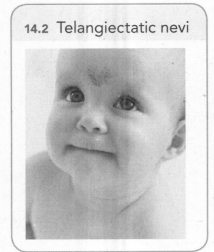

14.2 Telangiectatic nevi

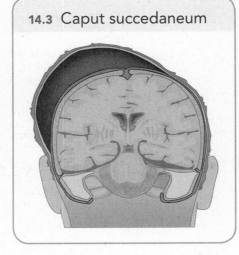

14.3 Caput succedaneum

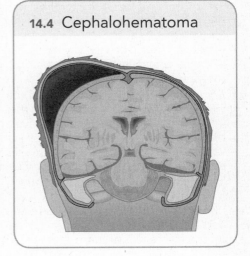

14.4 Cephalohematoma

Mouth

- Determine whether the palate is intact.
- Determine strength of sucking.
- Lip movements should be symmetrical.
- Saliva should be scant. Excessive saliva can indicate a tracheoesophageal fistula.
- Epstein pearls (small white cysts found on the gums and at the junction of the soft and hard palates) are expected findings. They result from the accumulation of epithelial cells and disappear a few weeks after birth.
- Tongue should move freely, be symmetrical in shape, and not protrude. (A protruding tongue can be an indication of Down syndrome.)
- Soft and hard palate should be intact.
- Gums and tongue should be pink. Gray-white patches on the tongue and gums can indicate thrush, a fungal infection caused by *Candida albicans*, sometimes acquired from the mother's vaginal secretions.

Neck

- Neck should be short, thick, surrounded by skin folds, and exhibit no webbing.
- Neck should move freely from side to side and up and down.
- Absence of head control can indicate prematurity or Down syndrome.

Chest

- Chest should be barrel-shaped.
- Respirations are primarily diaphragmatic.
- Clavicles should be intact.
- Absence of retractions.
- Nipples should be prominent, well formed, and symmetrical.
- Breast nodules can be 3 to 10 mm.

Abdomen

- Umbilical cord should be odorless and exhibit no intestinal structures.
- Abdomen should be round, dome-shaped, and nondistended.
- Bowel sounds should be present 1 to 2 hr following birth.

Anogenital

- Anus should be present, patent, and not covered by a membrane.
- Meconium should be passed within 48 hr after birth.
- Genitalia of a male newborn should include rugae on the scrotum.
- Testes should be present in the scrotum.
- Male urinary meatus is located at penile tip.
- Genitalia of a female should include labia majora covering the labia minora and clitoris, and is usually edematous.
- Vaginal blood-tinged discharge can occur in female newborns, which is caused by maternal pregnancy hormones. This is an expected finding.
- A hymenal tag should be present.
- Urine should be passed within 24 hr after birth. Uric acid crystals will produce a rust color in the urine the first couple of days of life.

Extremities

- Determine range of motion, symmetry of motion, and spontaneous movements.
- Extremities should be flexed.
- Observe for bowed legs and flat feet, which should be present because lateral muscles are more developed than the medial muscles.
- Gluteal folds should be symmetrical.
- Soles should be well-lined over two-thirds of the feet.
- Nail beds should be pink, and no extra digits are present.

Spine

Spine should be straight, flat, midline and easily flexed.

Reflexes

Sucking and rooting reflex
- EXPECTED FINDING: Elicit by stroking the cheek or edge of mouth. Newborn turns the head toward the side that is touched and starts to suck.
- EXPECTED AGE: Usually disappears after 3 to 4 months but can persist up to 1 year

Palmar grasp
- EXPECTED FINDING: Elicit by placing examiner's finger in palm of newborn's hand. The newborn's fingers curl around examiner's fingers.
- EXPECTED AGE: Lessens between 3 and 4 months

Plantar grasp
- EXPECTED FINDING: Elicit by placing examiner's finger at base of newborn's toes. The newborn responds by curling toes downward.
- EXPECTED AGE: Birth to 8 months

Moro reflex
- EXPECTED FINDING: Elicit by allowing the head and trunk of the newborn in a semisitting position to fall backward to an angle of at least 30°. The newborn will symmetrically extend and then abduct the arms at the elbows and fingers spread to form a "C."
- EXPECTED AGE: Birth to 6 months

Tonic neck reflex (fencing)
- EXPECTED FINDING: With newborn in supine, neutral position, examiner turns newborn's head quickly to one side. The newborn's arm and leg on that side extend and opposing arm and leg flex.
- EXPECTED AGE: Birth to 3 to 4 months

Babinski reflex (plantar)
- EXPECTED FINDING: Elicit by stroking outer edge of sole of the foot, moving up toward toes. Toes will fan upward and out. (14.5)
- EXPECTED AGE: Birth to 1 year

Stepping (walking)
- EXPECTED FINDING: Elicit by holding the newborn upright with feet touching a flat surface. The newborn responds with stepping movements.
- EXPECTED AGE: Birth to 4 weeks

Senses

Vision: The newborn should be able to focus on objects 8 to 12 inches away from face. This is approximately the distance from the mother's face when the newborn is breastfeeding. The eyes are sensitive to light, so newborns prefer dim lighting. Pupils are reactive to light, and the blink reflex is easily stimulated. The newborn can track high-contrast objects and prefers bright colors and patterns. Term newborns can see objects as far away as 2.5 feet. By the age of 3 months, they can discriminate colors.

Hearing: Hearing is similar to that of an adult once the amniotic fluid drains from the ears. Newborns exhibit selective listening to familiar voices and rhythms of intrauterine life. The newborn turns toward the general direction of a sound.

Touch: Newborns should respond to tactile messages of pain and touch. The mouth is the area most sensitive to touch in the newborn.

Taste: Newborns can taste and prefer sweet to salty, sour, or bitter.

Smell: Newborns have a highly developed sense of smell, prefer sweet smells, and can recognize the mother's smell.

Habitation: This is a protective mechanism whereby the newborn becomes accustomed to environmental stimuli. Response to a constant or repetitive stimulus is decreased. This allows the newborn to select stimuli that promotes continued learning, avoiding overload.

> **!** Reinforce teaching with the mother and family about the neonate's appearance, and give reassurance about expected findings that the family can be concerned about (milia, Epstein's pearls, caput succedaneum).

DIAGNOSTIC AND THERAPEUTIC PROCEDURES FOLLOWING BIRTH

Cord blood is collected at birth. Laboratory tests are conducted to determine ABO blood type and Rh status if the mother's blood type is O or she is Rh-negative. A CBC can be done by a capillary stick to evaluate for anemia, polycythemia, infection, or clotting problems. Blood glucose is done to evaluate for hypoglycemia.

EXPECTED LABORATORY VALUES

- **Hgb:** 14 to 24 g/dL
- **Platelets:** 150,000 to 300,000/mm³
- **Hct:** 44% to 64%
- **Glucose:** 40 to 60 mg/dL
- **RBC count:** 4.8 x 10⁶ to 7.1 x 10⁶
- **Bilirubin**
  - 24 hr: 2 to 6 mg/dL
  - 48 hr: 6 to 7 mg/dL
  - 3 to 5 days: 4 to 6 mg/dL
- **Leukocytes:** 9,000 to 30,000/mm³

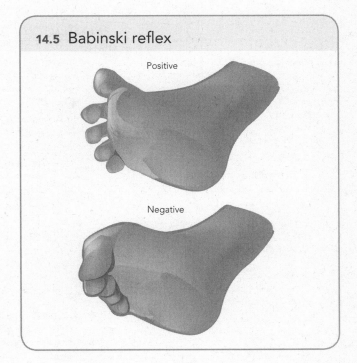

14.5 Babinski reflex

Positive

Negative

COMPLICATIONS

Airway obstruction related to mucus

NURSING ACTIONS: Suction mouth and nose with a bulb syringe. Gentle percussion over the chest can help loosen secretions.

Hypothermia

NURSING ACTIONS

- Monitor axillary temperature. Healthy newborn skin temperature is approximately 36.5° to 37° C (97.7° to 98.6° F)
- If temperature is unstable, place the newborn in a radiant warmer, and maintain skin temperature at approximately 36.5° C (97.7° F). Ideal method for promoting warmth and maintaining neonate's body temperature for a stable newborn is early skin-to-skin contact with the mother. If the infant does not remain skin-to-skin with the mother during the first 1 to 2 hr after birth, the nurse places the thoroughly dried infant under the radiant warmer or in a warm incubator until body temperature stabilizes.
- Monitor axillary temperature every hour until stable.
- All exams and data collection should be performed under a radiant warmer or during skin-to-skin contact with the mother.

Inadequate oxygen supply

Related to obstructed airway, poorly functioning cardiopulmonary system, or hypothermia

NURSING ACTIONS

- Monitor respirations and skin color for cyanosis.
- Stabilize the body temperature or clear airway as indicated, administer oxygen, and if needed, prepare for resuscitation.

Application Exercises

1. A nurse is caring for a newborn who was born at 38 weeks of gestation, weighs 3,200 g, and is in the 60th percentile for weight. Based on the weight and gestational age, the nurse should assign the newborn which of the following classifications?

   A. Low birth weight

   B. Appropriate for gestational age

   C. Small for gestational age

   D. Large for gestational age

2. A nurse is collecting data from a newborn and observes small white nodules on the roof of the newborn's mouth. This finding is a characteristic of which of the following conditions?

   A. Mongolian spots

   B. Milia spots

   C. Erythema toxicum

   D. Epstein pearls

3. A nurse is evaluating the reflexes of a newborn. In checking for the Moro reflex, the nurse should perform which of the following actions?

   A. Hold the newborn vertically under arms and allow one foot to touch table.

   B. Stimulate the pads of the newborn's hands with stroking or massage.

   C. Stimulate the soles of the newborn's feet on the outer lateral surface of each foot.

   D. Hold the newborn in a semi-sitting position, then allow the newborn's head and trunk to fall backward.

4. A nurse is collecting data from a newborn following birth. Which of the following findings indicate the newborn is adapting to extrauterine life? (Select all that apply.)

   A. Expiratory grunting

   B. Inspiratory nasal flaring

   C. Apnea for 10-second periods

   D. Obligate nasal breathing

   E. Crackles and wheezing

5. A nurse is reinforcing teaching with a new mother on bathing a newborn. The newborn has a bluish marking across the lower back. Which of the following statements should the nurse make concerning the variation?

   A. "This is frequently seen in newborns of African American, Asian, or Native American origin."

   B. "This is a finding indicating hyperbilirubinemia."

   C. "This is a forceps mark from an operative delivery."

   D. "This is related to prolonged birth or trauma during delivery."

PRACTICE Active Learning Scenario

A nurse in the nursery is assisting with admitting a newborn 2 hr following birth. What nursing actions should the nurse use to evaluate newborn physical development? Use the ATI Active Learning Template: Growth and Development to complete this item.

PHYSICAL DEVELOPMENT

- Describe at least three tools for data collection.
- Describe four reflex responses present at birth and how they are elicited.
- Describe newborn heart rate and how it is evaluated.

Application Exercises Key

1. A. A newborn who has a low birth weight would weigh less than 2,500 g.

   B. **CORRECT:** This newborn is classified as appropriate for gestational age because the weight is between the 10th and 90th percentile.

   C. A newborn who is small for gestational age would weigh less than the 10th percentile.

   D. A newborn who is large for gestational age would weigh greater than the 90th percentile.

   Ⓝ *NCLEX® Connection: Health Promotion and Maintenance, Data Collection Techniques*

2. A. Mongolian spots are dark areas observed in newborns of African American, Asian, or Native American origin.

   B. Milia are small white bumps that occur on the nose due to clogged sebaceous glands.

   C. Erythema toxicum is a transient maculopapular rash seen in newborns.

   D. **CORRECT:** Epstein's pearls are small white nodules that appear on the roof of a newborn's mouth.

   Ⓝ *NCLEX® Connection: Health Promotion and Maintenance, Data Collection Techniques*

3. A. Holding the newborn vertically under the arms and allowing one foot to touch the table elicits the stepping reflex.

   B. Stimulating the pads of the newborn's hands elicits the grasp reflex.

   C. Stimulating the outer lateral portion of the newborn's soles elicits the Babinski reflex.

   D. **CORRECT:** The Moro reflex is elicited by holding the newborn in a semi-sitting position and then allowing the head and trunk to fall backward.

   Ⓝ *NCLEX® Connection: Health Promotion and Maintenance, Data Collection Techniques*

4. A. Expiratory grunting is a manifestation of respiratory distress.

   B. Nasal flaring is a manifestation of respiratory distress.

   C. **CORRECT:** Periods of apnea lasting less than 15 seconds are an expected finding.

   D. **CORRECT:** Newborns are considered obligate nasal breathers.

   E. Crackles and wheezing are manifestations of fluid or infection in the lungs.

   Ⓝ *NCLEX® Connection: Health Promotion and Maintenance, Aging Process*

5. A. **CORRECT:** Mongolian spots are commonly found over the lumbosacral area of newborns who are of African American, Asian, or Native American origin.

   B. Hyperbilirubinemia would present as jaundice.

   C. Forceps marks would most likely present as a cephalohematoma.

   D. Birth trauma would present as ecchymosis.

   Ⓝ *NCLEX® Connection: Physiological Adaptation, Alterations in Body Systems*

PRACTICE Answer

Using the ATI Active Learning Template: Growth and Development

PHYSICAL DEVELOPMENT

Data collection tools
- Brief initial data collection of all systems
- Gestational age: Physical measurements and New Ballard Scale
- Vital signs
- Head-to-toe physical examination

Reflexes
- Sucking and rooting: Turns head to side that is touched and begins to suck when cheek or edge of mouth is stroked.
- Palmar grasp: Grasps object when placed in palm.
- Plantar grasp: Toes curl downward when sole of the foot is touched.
- Moro reflex: Arms and legs symmetrically extend and then abduct while fingers spread to form a "C" when infant's head and trunk are allowed to fall backward to an angle of at least 30°.
- Tonic neck (fencer position): Extends arm and leg on same side when head is turned to that side, and flexes arm and leg of opposite side.
- Babinski: Toes fan upward and out when outer edge of sole of foot is stroked, moving up toward toes.
- Stepping: Makes stepping movements when held upright with feet touching flat surface.

Heart rate
- 100 to 160/min with brief fluctuations above and below, depending on activity level.
- When newborn is sleeping, place pediatric stethoscope head on fourth or fifth intercostal space at the left midclavicular line over apex of the heart. Listen for 1 full minute.
- Note any murmurs.

Ⓝ *NCLEX® Connection: Health Promotion and Maintenance, Aging Process*

CHAPTER 15

CHAPTER 15 *Nursing Care of Newborns*

Nurses play an important role in the care of newborns after birth. Initial nursing care includes maintaining a patent airway, monitoring vital signs, ensuring proper identification, maintaining thermoregulation, monitoring elimination patterns, preventing infection, and reinforcing discharge teaching for parents.

Low-risk newborn

PATIENT-CENTERED CARE

NURSING CARE

- Vital signs should be checked on admission/birth, every 30 min × 2, every 1 hr × 2, and then every 8 hr.
- Weight should be checked shortly after birth once the newborn is stable, and daily at the same time using the same scale.
- Inspect the umbilical cord. Ensure that the cord is clamped securely to prevent hemorrhage.
- Using the facility's preferred pain assessment tool, monitor the client's pain every 8 to 12 hr and following painful procedures. Qᴘᴄᴄ

Respiratory system

INTERVENTIONS FOR STABILIZATION AND RESUSCITATION OF AIRWAY

- The newborn is able to clear most secretions in air passages by the cough reflex. Routine suctioning of the mouth, then the nasal passages with a bulb syringe, is done to remove excess mucus in the respiratory tract.
  ○ Compress bulb before insertion into one side of the mouth.
  ○ Avoid center of the mouth to prevent stimulating gag reflex.
  ○ Aspirate mouth first, one nostril, then second nostril.
- Newborns delivered by cesarean birth are more susceptible to fluid remaining in the lungs than newborns who were delivered vaginally.
- If bulb suctioning is unsuccessful, mechanical suction can be used, as well as the institution of emergency procedures.

Thermoregulation

Thermoregulation provides a neutral thermal environment that helps a newborn maintain a stable core temperature with minimal oxygen consumption and caloric expenditure. A newborn has a relatively large surface-to-weight ratio, reduced metabolism per unit area, blood vessels close to the surface, and small amounts of insulation.

- The newborn keeps warm by metabolizing brown fat, which is unique to newborns, but only within a very narrow temperature range. Becoming chilled (cold stress) can increase the newborn's oxygen demands and rapidly use up brown fat reserves. Therefore, monitoring temperature regulation is important.
- Monitor for hypothermia in the newborn.
  ○ Axillary temperature less than 36.5° C (97.7° F)
  ○ Cyanosis
  ○ Increased respiratory rate

INTERVENTIONS TO MAINTAIN THERMOREGULATION

- Core temperature varies within newborns but should be kept at approximately 36.5° to 37° C (97.7° to 98.6° F). Heat loss occurs by four mechanisms.
  ○ **Conduction:** Loss of body heat resulting from direct contact with a cooler surface.
    ▪ Preheat a radiant warmer.
    ▪ Warm a stethoscope and other instruments.
    ▪ Pad a scale before weighing the newborn.
    ▪ The newborn should be placed directly on the client's chest and covered with a warm blanket.
  ○ **Convection:** Flow of heat from the body surface to cooler environmental air.
    ▪ Place the bassinet out of the direct line of a fan or air conditioning vent.
    ▪ Swaddle the newborn in a blanket.
    ▪ Any procedure done with the newborn uncovered should be performed under a radiant heat source.
    ▪ Keep ambient temperature of the nursery or client's room at 22° to 26° C (72° to 78° F).
  ○ **Evaporation:** Loss of heat as surface liquid is converted to vapor.
    ▪ Gently rub the newborn dry with a warm sterile blanket (adhering to standard precautions) immediately after delivery.
    ▪ If thermoregulation is unstable, postpone the initial bath until the newborn's skin temperature is 36.5° C (97.7° F).
    ▪ When bathing, expose only one body part at a time, washing and drying thoroughly.
  ○ **Radiation:** Loss of heat from the body surface to a cooler solid surface that is close to, but not in direct contact. Keep the newborn and examining tables away from windows and air conditioners.
- Temperature stabilizes at 37° C (98.6° F) within 4 hr after birth if chilling is prevented.

Identification

Identification is applied to the newborn by the nurse immediately after birth. The nurse should ensure the information on the infant's and parent's bracelets matches exactly. It is an important safety measure to prevent the newborn from being given to the wrong parents, switched, or abducted. Qs

- The newborn, client, and client's partner are identified by plastic identification wristbands with permanent locks that must be cut to be removed. Identification bands should include the newborn's name, sex, date, and time of birth, and client's medical record number. The newborn should have one band placed on the ankle and one on the wrist. In addition, the newborn's footprints and client's finger print are taken. The above information is also included with the footprint sheet.
- Each time the newborn is given to the parents, the identification band should be verified against the client's identification band.
- All facility staff who assist in caring for the newborn are required to wear photo identification badges.
- The newborn is not to be given to anyone who does not have a photo identification badge that distinguishes that person as a staff member of the maternal-newborn unit.
- Many facilities have locked maternal-newborn units that require staff to permit entrance or exit. Some have a sensor device on the ID band or umbilical cord clamp that sounds an alarm if the newborn is removed from the facility.

Bathing

- The initial bath can be given once the newborn's temperature has stabilized to at least 36.5° C (97.7° F). A complete sponge bath should be given under a radiant heat source to prevent heat loss. If necessary, the first bath will be postponed until thermoregulation stabilizes.
- Gloves should be worn until after the newborn's first bath to avoid exposure to body secretions.

Infection control

Infection control is essential in preventing cross-contamination from newborn to newborn and between newborns and staff. Newborns are at risk for infection during the first few months of life due to immature immune systems.

- Provide individual bassinets equipped with a thermometer, diapers, T-shirts, and bathing supplies.
- All personnel who care for a newborn should scrub with antimicrobial soap from elbows to fingertips before entering the nursery. In between care of the newborn, the nurse should follow facility hygiene protocols.

MEDICATIONS

Erythromycin

- Prophylactic eye care involves mandatory instillation of antibiotic ointment into the eyes to prevent ophthalmia neonatorum.
- Infections can be transmitted during descent through the birth canal. Ophthalmia neonatorum is caused by *Neisseria gonorrhoeae* or *Chlamydia trachomatis* and can cause blindness.

NURSING ACTIONS
- Use a single-dose unit to avoid cross-contamination.
- Apply a 1 to 2 cm ribbon of ointment to the lower conjunctival sac of each eye, starting from the inner canthus and moving outward.
- A possible adverse effect is chemical conjunctivitis, causing redness, swelling, and drainage for 24 to 48 hr. Reassure the parents that this will resolve on its own.
- Application can be delayed for 1 hr after birth to facilitate bonding.

Vitamin K (phytonadione)

Administered to prevent hemorrhagic disorders. Vitamin K is not produced in the gastrointestinal tract of the newborn until around day 7. Vitamin K is produced in the colon by bacteria that forms once formula or breast milk is introduced into the gut of the newborn.

NURSING ACTIONS: Administer 0.5 to 1 mg intramuscularly into the vastus lateralis (where muscle development is adequate) within 1 hr after birth.

Hepatitis B immunization

Provides protection against hepatitis B

NURSING ACTIONS
- Recommended to be administered to all newborns.
- Informed consent must be obtained.
- For newborns born to healthy clients, recommended dosage schedule is at birth, 1 month, and 6 months.
- For clients infected with hepatitis B, hepatitis B immunoglobulin and the hepatitis B vaccine are given within 12 hr of birth. The hepatitis B vaccine is given alone at 1 month, 2 months, and 12 months.

! It is important **NOT** to give the vitamin K and the hepatitis B injections in the same thigh. Sites should be alternated.

LABORATORY TESTS

Cord blood for type and Rh immediately following delivery.

Blood glucose for hypoglycemia per facility policy or as prescribed

Metabolic screening
- Universal newborn screening is mandated in all states. A capillary heel stick should be done 24 hr following birth. For results to be accurate, the newborn must have received formula or breast milk for at least 24 hr. If the newborn is discharged before 24 hr of age, the test should be repeated in 1 to 2 weeks.
- All states require testing for phenylketonuria (PKU). PKU is a defect in protein metabolism in which the accumulation of the amino acid phenylalanine can result in mental retardation. (Treatment in the first 2 months of life can prevent mental retardation.)

Bilirubin level on all newborns prior to discharge.

Collecting blood samples
- Heelstick blood samples are obtained by the nurse, who dons clean gloves.
- Administer oral sucrose and offer a pacifier for pain management.
- Warm the heel first to increase circulation.
- Cleanse the area with an appropriate antiseptic, and allow for drying.
- A spring-activated lancet is used so that the skin incision is made quickly and painlessly.
- The outer aspect of the heel should be used, and the lancet should go no deeper than 2.4 mm to prevent necrotizing osteochondritis resulting from penetration of bone with the lancet.
- Follow facility protocol for specimen collection, equipment to be used, and labeling of specimens.
- Apply pressure with dry gauze (do not use alcohol because it will cause bleeding to continue) until bleeding stops, and cover with an adhesive bandage.
- Cuddle and comfort the newborn when the procedure is completed to reassure the newborn and promote feelings of safety.

DIAGNOSTIC PROCEDURES

Newborn hearing screening is required in most states. Newborns are screened so that hearing impairments can be detected and treated early. Q_EBP

COMPLICATIONS

Respiratory distress

Ineffective airway clearance following delivery or prematurity can lead to respiratory distress in the newborn.

NURSING ACTIONS: Monitor for manifestations of respiratory complications.
- Bradypnea: respirations less than or equal to 30/min
- Tachypnea: respirations greater than or equal to 60/min
- Abnormal breath sounds: expiratory grunting, crackles, wheezes
- Respiratory distress: nasal flaring, retractions, grunting, gasping, labored breathing

Cold stress

Ineffective thermoregulation can lead to hypoxia, acidosis, and hypoglycemia. Newborns who have respiratory distress are at a higher risk for hypothermia.

NURSING ACTIONS
- Monitor for manifestations of cold stress (cyanotic trunk, depressed respirations).
- The newborn should be warmed slowly over 2 to 4 hr. Correct hypoxia by administering oxygen. Correct acidosis and hypoglycemia. Q_EBP

Hypoglycemia

Frequently occurs in the first few hours of life secondary to the use of energy to establish respirations and maintain body heat
- Newborns who are small or large for gestational age, less than 37 weeks of gestation, greater than 42 weeks of gestation, or born to clients who have diabetes mellitus are at risk for hypoglycemia and should have blood glucose monitored within the first 2 hr of life.
- Follow facility protocols regarding frequency of monitoring blood glucose levels.

NURSING ACTIONS
- Monitor for jitteriness; twitching; weak, high-pitched cry; irregular respiratory effort; cyanosis; lethargy; eye rolling; seizures; and blood glucose level less than 40 mg/dL by heel stick.
- Have the client breastfeed immediately or give donor breast milk or formula to elevate blood glucose levels. Brain damage can result if brain cells are depleted of glucose.

Nutritional needs for the newborn

- Normal newborn weight loss immediately after birth and subsequent weight gain should be as follows.
  - **Loss of 5% to 10% after birth (regain 10 to 14 days after birth)**
  - **Gain of 110 to 200 g/week for first 3 months**
- Healthy newborns need a fluid intake of 100 to 140 mL/kg/24 hr. Newborns do not need to be given water because they receive sufficient water from breast milk or formula.
- Adequate caloric intake is essential to provide energy for growth, digestion, metabolic needs, and activity. For the first 3 months, the newborn requires 110 kcal/kg/day. From 3 to 6 months, the requirement decreases to 100 kcal/kg/day. Both breast milk and formula provide 20 kcal/oz.
- Carbohydrates should make up 40% to 50% of the newborn's total caloric intake. The most abundant carbohydrate in breast milk or formula is lactose.
- At least 15% of calories must come from fat (triglycerides). The fat in breast milk is easier to digest than the fat in cow's milk.
- For adequate growth and development, a newborn must receive 2.25 to 4 g/kg/day of protein.
- Breast milk contains the vitamins necessary to provide adequate newborn nutrition.
- The mineral content of commercial newborn formula and breast milk is adequate with the exception of iron and fluoride.
  - Iron is low in all forms of milk, but it is absorbed better from breast milk. Newborns who only breastfeed for the first 6 months maintain adequate hemoglobin levels and do not need additional iron supplementation. After 6 months of age, all newborns need to be fed iron-fortified cereal and other foods rich in iron. Newborns who are formula-fed should receive iron-fortified newborn formula until 12 months of age. Clients who breastfeed their newborns are encouraged to do so for the newborn's first 12 months of life.
  - Fluoride levels in breast milk and formulas are low. A fluoride supplement should be given to newborns not receiving fluoridated water after 6 months of age.
- Solids are not introduced until 6 months of age. If introduced too early, food allergies can develop.
- A client's preference on the type of feeding to offer the newborn is influenced by prior experience, knowledge of options, culture, physical and physiological conditions, emotions, and views of the client's support system. Qpcc

ADVANTAGES OF BREASTFEEDING

BENEFITS OF BREASTFEEDING

- Reduces the risk of infection by providing IgA antibodies, lysozymes, leukocytes, macrophages, and lactoferrin that prevents infections
- Promotes rapid brain growth due to large amounts of lactose
- Provides protein and nitrogen for neurological cell building and improves the newborn's ability to regulate calcium and phosphorus levels
- Contains electrolytes and minerals
- Easy for the newborn to digest
- Convenient and inexpensive
- Reduces incidence of sudden infant death syndrome (SIDS), allergies, asthma, otitis media, diabetes mellitus, and obesity throughout life
- Promotes maternal-infant bonding and attachment

NURSING INTERVENTIONS

Successful breastfeeding

- Place the newborn skin-to-skin on the client's chest immediately after birth. Initiate breastfeeding as soon as possible or within the first 30 min following birth.
- Explain breastfeeding techniques to the client. Have the client wash her hands, get comfortable, and have caffeine-free fluids to drink during breastfeeding.
- Reassure the client that uterine cramps are normal during breastfeeding, resulting from oxytocin, which also promote uterine involution.
- Express a few drops of colostrum or milk and spread it over the nipple to lubricate the nipple and entice the newborn.
- Show the client the proper latch-on position. Have her support the breast in one hand with the thumb on top and four fingers underneath. With the newborn's mouth in front of the nipple, the newborn can be stimulated to open his mouth by tickling his lower lip with the tip of the nipple. The client pulls the newborn to the nipple with his mouth covering part of the areola as well as the nipple.
- Explain to the client that when the newborn is latched on correctly, his nose, cheeks, and chin will be touching her breast. Hunger cues include hand-to-mouth or hand-to-hand movements, sucking motions, and rooting reflex.
- Demonstrate the four basic breastfeeding positions: football hold (under the arm), cradle (most common), modified cradle (across the lap), and side-lying. **(15.1)**
- Encourage the client to breastfeed at least 15 to 20 min per breast to ensure that the newborn receives adequate fat and protein.
- Explain to the client that newborns will nurse on demand after a pattern is established and that the amount of milk the breast produces is dependent on the frequency and length of feedings.
- Show the client how to insert a finger in the side of the newborn's mouth to break the suction from the nipple prior to removing the newborn from the breast to prevent nipple trauma.
- Show the client how to burp the newborn when alternating breasts. The newborn should be burped either over the shoulder or in an upright position with the chin supported. The client should gently pat the newborn on the back to elicit a burp.
- Tell the client to begin the next feeding with the breast she stopped feeding with in the previous feeding.

- Offer referral to breastfeeding support groups. Q_{TC}
- Contact a lactation consultant to offer additional recommendations and support, especially to clients who have concerns about adequate breast milk or clients who have been unsuccessful with breastfeeding in the past.
- Inform the client how to tell if the newborn is receiving adequate feeding (gaining weight, voiding six to eight diapers per day, and contentedness between feedings).

CLIENT EDUCATION
- The newborn can have loose, pale, and yellow stools during breastfeeding. This is normal.
- Avoid nipple confusion in the newborn by not offering supplemental formula, pacifier, or soothers until breastfeeding has been established, typically in 2 to 3 weeks. Supplementation can be provided using a small cup or syringe feeding, if needed. When supplementation is deemed necessary, giving the baby expressed breast milk is best.
- Herbal products, such as fenugreek or blessed thistle, and prescription medications, such as metoclopramide, have been reported to increase breast milk production. There is insufficient data to confirm or deny their effect on lactation. Check with the provider before taking over-the-counter or prescription medications. Q_{EBP}

Successful storage of breast milk obtained by a breast pump

CLIENT EDUCATION
- Breast milk can still be provided to the newborn during periods of separation by using a breast pump or hand expression.
  - Breast pumps can be manual, electric, or battery-operated and pumped directly into a bottle or freezer bag.
  - One or both breasts can be pumped, and suction is adjustable for comfort.
- Breast milk must be stored according to guidelines for proper containers, labeling, refrigerating, and freezing.
  - Breast milk can be stored at room temperature under very clean conditions for up to 8 hr. It can be refrigerated in sterile bottles for use within 8 days, or can be frozen in sterile containers in the freezer compartment of a refrigerator for up to 6 months. Breast milk can be stored in a deep freezer for 12 months.
  - Thawing the milk in the refrigerator for 24 hr is the best way to preserve the immunoglobulins present in it. It also can be thawed by holding the container under running lukewarm water or placing it in a container of lukewarm water. The bottle should be rotated often, but not shaken when thawing in this manner.
  - Thawing by microwave is contraindicated because it destroys some of the immune factors and lysozymes contained in the milk. Microwave thawing also leads to the development of hot spots in the milk because of uneven heating, which can burn the newborn.
  - Do not refreeze thawed milk.
  - Used portions of breast milk must be discarded.

15.1 Breastfeeding positions

Football hold

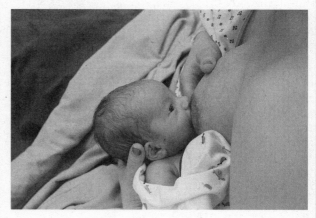

Cradle

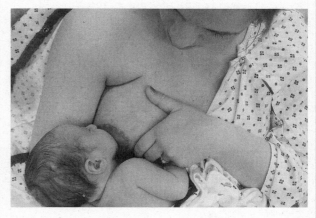

Modified cradle

The mother positions the baby as in the cradle position shown above, but reverses the function of each arm.

Side-lying

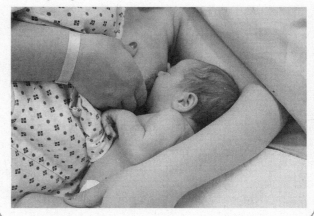

HUMAN MILK FEEDING/DONOR MILK

If the client is not able to provide the breast milk, the recommended alternative is pasteurized donor milk from a milk bank. (Obtain informed consent.) However, in many cases, it's not readily accessible, and a commercial infant formula is used.

FORMULA (BOTTLE) FEEDING

Formula can be a successful and adequate source of nutrition if the client does not breastfeed. The newborn should be fed every 3 to 4 hr. Parents should awaken the newborn to feed at least every 3 hr during the day and at least every 4 hr during the night until the newborn is feeding well and gaining weight adequately. Then, a feed-on-demand schedule can be followed.

NURSING INTERVENTIONS

- Reinforce teaching with the parents about how to prepare formula (mix according to instructions), bottles, and nipples. Review the importance of hand washing prior to formula preparation.
- Reinforce teaching with the parents about the different forms of formula (ready-to-feed, concentrated, powder) and how to prepare each correctly.
- Reinforce teaching with the parents about how to tell if their newborn is being adequately fed (gaining weight; bowel movements are yellow, soft and formed; and satisfaction between feedings). Breastfed infants usually have 3 or more bowel movements a day; formula-fed infants less frequent. Breastfed and formula-fed infants usually have 6 or more wet diapers a day.

CLIENT EDUCATION

- Bottles and accessories can be put in the dishwasher, boiled, or washed by hand in hot soapy water using a good bottle and nipple brush.
- Wash the lid of a can of concentrated formula with hot, soapy water. Shake before opening it.
- Use tap water to mix concentrated or powder formula. If the water source is questionable, tap water should be boiled first.
- Prepared formula can be refrigerated for up to 48 hr.
- Check the flow of formula from the bottle to ensure it is not coming out too slow or too fast.
- Do not to use formula past the expiration date on the container.
- Cradle the newborn in the arms in a semi-upright position. Do not place the newborn in the supine position during bottle feeding because of the danger of aspiration. Newborns who bottle feed do best when held close and at a 45° angle.
- Place the nipple on top of the newborn's tongue.
- Keep the nipple filled with formula to prevent the newborn from swallowing air.
- Always hold the bottle and never prop the bottle for feeding.
- Give the newborn opportunities to burp several times during a feeding
- Discard any unused formula remaining in the bottle when the newborn is finished feeding due to the possibility of bacterial contamination. Qs

MONITORING NEWBORN FOR ADEQUATE GROWTH

- Monitor the newborn for adequate growth and weight gain.
  - Weights are taken daily in the newborn nursery. Growth is monitored by placing the newborn's weight on a growth chart. Adequate growth should be within the 10th to 90th percentile. Falling below the 10th percentile can indicate inadequate weight gain; above 90th percentile indicates excessive weight gain.
  - The newborn's length and head circumference are also routinely monitored and plotted on a growth chart to identify trends.
- Monitor the client's ability to feed the newborn, whether by breast or bottle.

RISK FACTORS FOR IMPAIRED NEWBORN NUTRITION

Risk factors for failure to thrive (newborn) can be related to ineffective feeding patterns or inadequate breastfeeding by the newborn or client.

NEWBORN FACTORS
- Inadequate breastfeeding
- Illness/infection
- Malabsorption
- Other conditions that increase energy needs

MATERNAL FACTORS
- Inadequate or slow milk production
- Inadequate emptying of the breast
- Inappropriate timing of feeding
- Inadequate breast tissue
- Pain with feeding
- Maternal hemorrhage
- Illness/infection

COMPLICATIONS FOR NEWBORN NUTRITION

There can be special considerations when a newborn has difficulty receiving adequate nutrition. Nursing interventions can often help these newborns receive adequate nutrition.

NEWBORNS WHO ARE SLEEPY
- Unwrap the newborn.
- Change the newborn's diaper.
- Hold the newborn upright, and turn him from side to side.
- Talk to the newborn.
- Massage the newborn's back, and rub his hands and feet.
- Apply a cool cloth to the newborn's face.

NEWBORNS WHO ARE FUSSY
- Swaddle the newborn.
- Hold the newborn close. Move and rock him gently.
- Reduce environmental stimuli.
- Place the newborn skin-to-skin.

Failure to thrive

Failure to thrive is slow weight gain, usually below the 5th percentile on the growth chart.

NEWBORNS WHO ARE BREASTFEEDING

- Evaluate positioning and latch during breastfeeding. **(15.1)**
- Massage the breast during feeding. **Q**EBP
- Determine feeding patterns and length of feedings.
- If the newborn is spitting up, the newborn can have an allergy to dairy products. Determine maternal intake of dairy products. The client might need to eliminate dairy from her diet. Instruct her to consume other food sources high in calcium or calcium supplements.

NEWBORNS WHO ARE FORMULA FEEDING

- Evaluate how much and how often the newborn is feeding.
- If the newborn is spitting up or vomiting, he can have an allergy or intolerance to cow's milk-based formula and can require a soy-based formula.

Nursing care and discharge teaching

- Prior to discharge, provide anticipatory guidance to prepare new parents to care for their newborn at home. Information should include causes of crying in the newborn, quieting techniques, sleeping patterns, hunger cues, feeding, and bathing the newborn.
- Parents need to be aware of the importance of well-baby checkups, immunization schedules, and when to call the provider for indications of illness.
- Stress providing a safe protective environment at home to new parents, including proper car seat usage, which is a very important part of the discharge instruction process. **Q**s
- Foster sibling interaction in newborn care

DETERMINATION OF FAMILY READINESS FOR HOME CARE OF THE NEWBORN

- Previous newborn experience and knowledge
- Parent-newborn attachment
- Adjustment to the parental role
- Social support
- Educational needs
- Sibling rivalry issues
- Readiness of the parents to have their home and lifestyle altered to accommodate their newborn
- Parents' ability to verbalize and demonstrate newborn care following instruction

INTERVENTIONS FOR HOME CARE OF THE NEWBORN

Through verbal discussion, pamphlets, and demonstration, provide education to the client and family regarding newborn behavior, quieting techniques, newborn care, indications of newborn wellbeing and illness, and issues of newborn safety. **Q**PCC

CRYING

Newborns cry when they are hungry, overstimulated, wet, cold, hot, tired, bored, or need to be burped. Assure the parents that, in time, they will learn what the newborn's cry means.

CLIENT EDUCATION

- Do not feed the newborn every time he cries. Overfeeding can lead to stomach aches and diarrhea.
- After checking the newborn, it is okay to let her cry for short periods of time.

QUIETING TECHNIQUES

- Swaddling
- Close skin contact
- Nonnutritive sucking with pacifier
- Rhythmic noises to simulate utero sounds
- Movement (a car ride, vibrating chair, infant swing, rocking newborn)
- Placing the newborn on his stomach across a holder's lap while gently bouncing legs
- En face position for eye contact (when parents and newborns faces are about 30 cm [12 in] apart and on the same plane)
- Stimulation

SLEEP-WAKE CYCLE

- Placing the newborn in the supine position for sleeping greatly decreases the risk of SIDS.
- Newborns sleep approximately 16 to 19 hr/day with periods of wakefulness gradually increasing.
- Many parents believe that adding solid food to the newborn's diet will help with sleep patterns. During the first 6 months of life, the American Academy of Pediatrics recommends only breastfeeding.
- Keep the environment quiet and dark at night.
- When awake, the newborn can be placed on his abdomen to promote muscle development for crawling. The infant should be supervised.
  - For nighttime feedings and diaper changes, keep a small night-light on to avoid having to turn on bright lights. Speak softly, and handle the newborn gently so that he goes back to sleep easily.
  - No bumper pads, loose linens, or toys should be placed in the bassinet.
  - Parents should sleep in close proximity but not in a shared space. Higher incidence rates are noted for SIDS and suffocation with bed sharing/co-sleeping.

ORAL AND NASAL SUCTIONING

Review correct technique with the parents.

POSITIONING AND HOLDING OF THE NEWBORN (HEAD SUPPORT)

Reinforce that the newborn has minimal head control. The head should be supported when the newborn is lifted because the head is larger and heavier than the rest of the body.

FOUR BASIC WAYS TO HOLD THE NEWBORN

- **Cradle hold:** Cradle the newborn's head in the bend of the elbow. This permits eye-to-eye contact and is a good position for feeding.
- **Upright position:** Hold the newborn upright. Face him toward the holder while supporting his head, upper back, and buttocks.
- **Football hold:** Support half of the newborn's body in the holder's forearm with the newborn's head and neck resting in the palm of the hand. This is a good position for breastfeeding and when shampooing the newborn's hair.
- **Colic hold:** Place the newborn face-down along the holder's forearm with the hand firmly between the newborn's legs. The newborn's cheek should be by the holder's elbow on the outside. The newborn should be able to see the ground. The holder's arm should be close to the body, using it to brace and steady the newborn. This is a good position for quieting a fussy newborn.

SWADDLING

Parents should be shown how to swaddle their newborn. Swaddling the newborn snugly in a receiving blanket helps the newborn feel more secure. Swaddling brings the newborn's extremities in closer to his trunk, which is similar to the intrauterine position. Q EBP

BATHING

- After the initial bath, the newborn's face, diaper area, and skin folds are cleansed daily. Complete bathing is performed two to three times per week using a mild soap that does not contain hexachlorophene.
- Bathing by immersion is not done until the newborn's umbilical cord has fallen off and the circumcision has healed.
  - Wash the area around the cord, taking care not to get the cord wet.
  - Move from the cleanest to dirtiest part of the newborn's body, beginning with the eyes, face, and head. Proceed to the chest, arms, and legs. Wash the groin area last.
- Reinforce proper newborn bathing techniques through a demonstration. Have the parents return the demonstration.
- Bathing should take place at the convenience of the parents, but not immediately after feeding to prevent spitting up and vomiting.
- Organize all equipment so that the newborn is not left unattended. Never leave the newborn alone in the tub or sink.
- Make sure the hot water heater is set at 49° C (120.2° F) or less. The room should be warm, and the bath water should be 38° C (100.4° F).
- Avoid drafts or chilling of the newborn. Expose only the body part being bathed, and dry the newborn thoroughly to prevent chilling and heat loss.

- Wrap the newborn in a towel, and swaddle him in a football hold to shampoo his head. Rinse shampoo from the newborn's head, and dry to avoid chilling.
- In male newborns, to cleanse an uncircumcised penis, wash with soap and water and rinse the penis. The foreskin should not be forced back or constriction can result.
- In female newborns, wash the vulva by wiping from front to back to prevent contamination of the vagina or urethra from rectal bacteria.
- Applying a fragrance-free, hypoallergenic, moisturizing emollient immediately after bathing can help prevent dry skin.
- Parents should dress the child in soft, temperature-appropriate clothing, covering the head when in cool temperatures.

FEEDING/ELIMINATION

- Clients who are breastfeeding should be seen by the lactation consultant.
- Newborns need to be breastfed on demand, at least 8 to 12 times in 24 hr. Newborns who are formula-fed should also be fed on demand or every 3 to 4 hr. Parents should awaken the newborn to feed at least every 3 hr during the day and at least every 4 hr at night.
- Clients should observe the newborn for feeding cues which indicate hunger, and provide a feeding when these are noted (hand-to-mouth or hand-to-hand movements, sucking motions, rooting, mouthing).
- Most newborns spit up a small amount after feedings. Keep the newborn upright and quiet for a few minutes after feedings.
- Breastfed newborns should have three or more bowel movements per day; bowel movements of formula fed newborns are less frequent. Regardless of the type of feeding used, all newborns should have six or more wet diapers per day.
  - The stools of newborns who are breastfed can appear yellow and seedy. They should have at least three stools per day for the first month. These stools are lighter in color and looser than the stools of newborns who are formula-fed.

DIAPERING

To avoid diaper rash, the newborn's diaper area should be kept clean and dry. Diapers should be changed frequently, and the perineal area cleaned with warm water or wipes and dried thoroughly to prevent skin breakdown. Diaper wipes with alcohol should be avoided.

CORD CARE

- Before discharge, the cord clamp is removed.
- Prevent cord infection by keeping the cord dry, and keep the top of the diaper folded down to expose the cord stump to air.
- Cord infection (a complication of improper cord care) can result if the cord is not kept clean and dry.
  - Monitor for manifestations of a cord that is moist and red, has a foul odor, or has purulent drainage.
  - Notify the provider immediately if findings of cord infection are present.

CIRCUMCISION CARE

Circumcision is the surgical removal of the foreskin of the penis.

- Circumcision is a personal choice made by the newborn's family for reasons of health and hygiene, religious conviction (Jewish male on eighth day after birth), tradition, culture, or social norms. Parents should make a well-informed decision in consultation with the provider.
- Circumcision should not be done immediately following birth because the newborn's level of vitamin K is at a low point, and the newborn would be at risk for hemorrhage.

HEALTH BENEFITS OF CIRCUMCISION

- Easier hygiene
- Decreased risk of urinary tract infections
- Decreased risk of STIs, including HIV
- Prevention of penile problems, such as phimosis
- Decreased risk of penile cancer and cervical cancer in female partners. Qᴘᴄᴄ

CONTRAINDICATIONS FOR CIRCUMCISION

- Newborns born with hypospadias (abnormal positioning of urethra on ventral undersurface of the penis) and epispadias (urethral canal terminates on dorsum of penis) because the prepuce skin can be needed for surgical repair of the defect
- Family history of bleeding disorders
- Newborns who are circumcised and whose parents decline vitamin K can be more likely to experience bleeding at the circumcision site, especially if they are breastfed.

Diagnostic and therapeutic procedures and management

ANESTHESIA: Anesthesia is required for circumcision. Types of anesthesia include a ring block, dorsal penile nerve block, topical anesthetic (eutectic mixture of local anesthetics), and concentrated oral sucrose. Nonpharmacologic methods, such as swaddling and nonnutritive sucking can be used to enhance pain management.

EQUIPMENT: Gomco (Yellen) or Mogen clamp, or Plastibell device

- The provider applies the Gomco (Yellen) or Mogen clamp to the penis, loosens the foreskin, and inserts the cone under the foreskin to provide a cutting surface for removal of the foreskin and to protect the penis. The wound is covered with sterile petroleum gauze to prevent infection and control bleeding.
- The provider slides the Plastibell device between the foreskin and the glans of the penis. The provider ties a suture tightly around the foreskin at the coronal edge of the glans. This applies pressure as the excess foreskin is removed from the penis. After 5 to 7 days, the Plastibell drops off, leaving a clean, healed excision. No petroleum is used for circumcision with the Plastibell. **(15.2)**

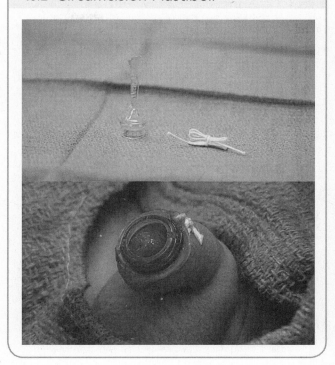

15.2 Circumcision Plastibell

Preprocedure

NURSING ACTIONS

- The newborn should be checked for the following.
  - A history of bleeding tendencies in the family (hemophilia and clotting disorders)
  - Hypospadias or epispadias
  - Ambiguous genitalia (genitalia that can include both male and female characteristics)
  - Illness or infection
- Signed informed consent form from parents is needed.
- Gather and prepare supplies.
- Administer prophylactic analgesia to newborn.
- Assist with procedure.
  - Place the newborn on the restraining board, and provide a radiant heat source to prevent cold stress. Do not leave the newborn unattended. Have bulb syringe readily available.
  - Comfort the newborn as needed.
  - Document time and type of circumcision, excessive bleeding, and voiding following procedure.

Postprocedure

NURSING ACTIONS

- Remove the newborn from the restraining board, and swaddle to provide comfort.
- Monitor for bleeding and voiding per facility protocol. Apply gauze lightly to the penis if bleeding or oozing is observed.
  - Bleeding every 15 to 30 min for the first hour and then hourly for the next 4 to 6 hr
  - The first voiding
- Fanfold diapers to prevent pressure on the circumcised area.

PARENT TEACHING

- The newborn will not be able to be bottle feed for 2 to 3 hr prior to the procedure to prevent vomiting and aspiration based on the preferences of the provider. Newborns who are breastfed can nurse up until the procedure.
- Keep the area clean. Change the newborn's diaper at least every 4 hr, and clean the penis with warm water with each diaper change. With clamp procedures, apply petroleum jelly with each diaper change for at least 24 hr after the circumcision to keep the diaper from adhering to the penis.
- A tub bath should not be given until the circumcision is healed. Until then, warm water should be trickled gently over the penis.
- Notify the provider if there is any redness, discharge, swelling, strong odor, tenderness, decrease in urination, or excessive crying from the newborn.
- A film of yellowish mucus can form over the glans by day two, and it is important not to wash it off.
- Avoid using premoistened towelettes to clean the penis because they contain alcohol.
- The newborn can be fussy or can sleep for several hours after the circumcision. Provide comfort measures for 24 to 48 hr.
- The circumcision will heal completely within a couple of weeks.

Complications and nursing management

Hemorrhage

- Monitor the newborn for bleeding.
- Provide gentle pressure on the penis using a small gauze square. If bleeding persists, notify the provider. Have a nurse continue to hold pressure until the provider arrives while another nurse prepares the circumcision tray and suture material.

Cold stress/hypoglycemia

- Monitor the newborn for excessive loss of heat resulting in increased respirations and lowered body temperature.
- Swaddle and feed the newborn as soon as the procedure is over.

Other complications

- Report any frank bleeding, foul-smelling drainage, or absence of voiding to the provider.
- Provide discharge instructions to the parents about manifestations of infection, comfort measures, medications, and when to notify the provider.

HOME SAFETY

- Never leave the newborn unattended with pets or other small children.
- Never leave the newborn alone on a bed, couch, or table. Newborns move enough to reach the edge and fall off.
- Never place the newborn on his stomach to sleep during the first few months of life. The back-lying position is the position of choice. The newborn can be placed on his abdomen when awake and being supervised.
- Never provide a newborn with a soft surface to sleep on (pillows or water bed). The newborn's mattress should be firm. Never put pillows, toys, bumper pads, or loose blankets in a crib. Crib linens should be tight-fitting.
- Do not tie anything around the newborn's neck.
- Monitor the safety of the newborn's crib. The space between the mattress and sides of the crib should be less than 2 fingerbreadths. The slats on the crib should be no more than 5.7 cm (2.25 in) apart.
- The newborn's crib or playpen should be away from window blinds and drapery cords. Newborns can become strangled in them.
- The bassinet or crib should be placed on an inner wall (not next to a window) to prevent cold stress by radiation.
- If an infant carrier is placed on a high place, such as a table, an adult should always be within arm's reach.
- Smoke detectors should be on every floor of a home and should be checked monthly to ensure that they are working.
- Eliminate potential fire hazards. Keep a crib and playpen away from heaters, radiators, and heat vents. Linens could catch fire if they come into contact with heat sources.
- Control the temperature and humidity of the newborn's environment by providing adequate ventilation.
- Avoid exposing the newborn to cigarette smoke in a home or elsewhere. Secondhand exposure increases the newborn's risk of developing respiratory illnesses.
- All visitors should wash their hands before touching the newborn. Any individual who has an infection should be kept away from the newborn.
- Carefully handle the newborn to prevent injury.
- Provide community resources to clients who can need additional and ongoing monitoring and instruction on newborn care (adolescent parents).

CAR SEAT SAFETY

Use an approved rear-facing car seat in the back seat, preferably in the middle (away from air bags and side impact) to transport the newborn. Keep infants in rear-facing car seats until age 2 or until the child reaches the maximum height and weight for the seat.

NEWBORN WELLNESS CHECKUPS

- Every newborn should be seen and examined at the doctor's office within 72 hr (3 days) after discharge. Wellness checkups should be scheduled per the recommendation of the pediatrician.
- Review the schedule for immunizations with the parents. Stress the importance of receiving these immunizations on a schedule for the newborn to be protected against diphtheria, tetanus, pertussis, hepatitis B, *Haemophilus influenzae*, polio, measles, mumps, rubella, influenza, rotavirus, pneumococcal, and varicella.

MANIFESTATIONS OF ILLNESS TO REPORT

Instruct parents regarding the manifestations of illness and to report them immediately.
- A temperature greater than 38° C (100.4° F) or less than 36.6° C (97.9° F)
- Poor feeding or little interest in food
- Forceful vomiting or frequent vomiting
- Decreased urination
- Diarrhea or decreased bowel movements
- Labored breathing with flared nostrils or an absence of breathing for greater than 15 seconds

- Jaundice
- Cyanosis
- Lethargy
- Inconsolable crying
- Difficulty waking
- Bleeding or purulent drainage around umbilical cord or circumcision
- Drainage developing in eyes

CARDIOPULMONARY RESUSCITATION

Encourage parents to seek CPR training.

PRACTICE Active Learning Scenario

A nurse is assisting with a class for parents on care of the newborn. What information should the nurse include in this class? Use the ATI Active Learning Template: Basic Concept to complete this item.

UNDERLYING PRINCIPLES: Describe three mechanisms that promote airway clearance.

NURSING INTERVENTIONS: Describe appropriate bulb syringe technique.

Application Exercises

1. A nurse is preparing to administer prophylactic eye ointment to a newborn to prevent ophthalmia neonatorum. Which of the following medications should the nurse anticipate administering?
   - A. Ofloxacin
   - B. Nystatin
   - C. Erythromycin
   - D. Ceftriaxone

2. A nurse is returning a newborn to his mother following circumcision. Which of the following actions should the nurse take to ensure safety of the newborn?
   - A. Ask the mother to state her full name.
   - B. Verify the name on the newborn's crib.
   - C. Match the mother's identification band with the newborn's band.
   - D. Confirm the mother's room number written on the crib.

3. A nurse is reinforcing teaching about breastfeeding with the mother of a newborn. Which of the following actions indicates understanding of the teaching?
   - A. The mother places a few drops of water on her nipple before beginning the feeding.
   - B. The mother ends the feeding by gently pulling her breast away from the newborn's mouth
   - C. When she is ready to breastfeed, the mother gently strokes the newborn's neck with her finger.
   - D. When latched on, the infant's nose, cheek, and chin are touching the mother's breast.

4. A nurse is reinforcing teaching about proper techniques for bottle feeding with a new mother. Which of the following instructions should the nurse provide?
   - A. Avoid burping the newborn until after the feeding.
   - B. Hold the newborn close in a supine position.
   - C. Keep the nipple full of formula throughout the feeding.
   - D. Refrigerate any formula left in the bottle.

5. A nurse is caring for a newborn. Which of the following actions by the newborn indicates readiness to feed?
   - A. Spits up clear mucus
   - B. Attempts to place his hand in his mouth
   - C. Turns his head toward sounds
   - D. Lies quietly with eyes open

6. A nurse is discussing circumcision with a newly hired nurse. Which of the following conditions should the nurse identify as contraindications? (Select all that apply.)
   - A. Hypospadias
   - B. Hydrocele
   - C. Family history of hemophilia
   - D. Hyperbilirubinemia
   - E. Epispadias

1. A. Ofloxacin is an antibiotic, but it is not used for ophthalmia neonatorum.

    B. Nystatin is used to treat *Candida albicans*, an oral yeast infection.

    C. **CORRECT:** One medication of choice for ophthalmia neonatorum is erythromycin ophthalmic ointment 0.5%. This antibiotic provides prophylaxis against *Neisseria gonorrhoeae* and *Chlamydia trachomatis*.

    D. Ceftriaxone is an antibiotic, but it is not used for ophthalmia neonatorum.

    Ⓝ *NCLEX® Connection: Pharmacological Therapies, Medication Administration*

2. A. Asking the mother to state her full name is not appropriate verification because two identifiers should be used.

    B. Looking at the name on the bassinet is not appropriate verification because two identifiers should be used.

    C. **CORRECT:** Each time the newborn is taken to the mother, the mother's identification band should be verified against the newborn's identification band.

    D. Confirming the mother's room number on the bassinet is not appropriate verification because it does not include two unique identifiers involving the mother and newborn.

    Ⓝ *NCLEX® Connection: Safety and Infection Control, Security Plan*

3. A. The infant is enticed to suck when the mother spreads colostrum on the nipple.

    B. The mother should insert a finger in the side of the newborn's mouth to break the suction before removing her nipple.

    C. The mother should stroke the newborn's lips with her nipple to promote sucking.

    D. **CORRECT:** Effective latching-on includes the infant's nose, cheek and chin touching the mother's breast.

    Ⓝ *NCLEX® Connection: Health Promotion and Maintenance, Ante/ Intra/Postpartum and Newborn Care*

4. A. The newborn should be burped after each ½ oz of formula.

    B. The newborn should be cradled in a semi-upright position.

    C. **CORRECT:** The nipple should always be kept full of formula to prevent the newborn from sucking in air during the feeding.

    D. Any formula left in the bottle should be discarded due to the possibility of bacterial contamination.

    Ⓝ *NCLEX® Connection: Health Promotion and Maintenance, Ante/ Intra/Postpartum and Newborn Care*

5. A. Spitting up, coughing, or gagging on mucus is an attempt by the newborn to clear his airway.

    B. **CORRECT:** Readiness-to-feed cues include the newborn making hand-to-mouth and hand-to-hand movements, sucking motions, rooting, and mouthing.

    C. The infant turns his head toward sounds in the environment as a sensory response indicating normal central nervous system functioning.

    D. Lying quietly with eyes open is an alerting behavior, indicating normal newborn reactivity.

    Ⓝ *NCLEX® Connection: Health Promotion and Maintenance, Ante/ Intra/Postpartum and Newborn Care*

6. A. **CORRECT:** Hypospadias involves a defect in the location of the urethral opening and is a contraindication to circumcision.

    B. Hydrocele, a collection of fluid in the scrotal sac, is not a contraindication to circumcision.

    C. **CORRECT:** A family history of hemophilia is a contraindication for circumcision.

    D. Hyperbilirubinemia is not a contraindication for circumcision.

    E. **CORRECT:** Epispadias involves a defect in the location of the urethral opening and is a contraindication to circumcision.

    Ⓝ *NCLEX® Connection: Reduction of Risk Potential, Potential for Complications of Diagnostic Tests/Treatments/Procedures*

PRACTICE Answer

Using the ATI Active Learning Template: Basic Concept

UNDERLYING PRINCIPLES: Mechanisms that promote airway clearance
- Infant's cough reflex
- Mechanical suctioning, back blows/chest thrusts
- Use of the bulb syringe for suctioning

NURSING INTERVENTIONS: Bulb syringe technique
- Depress the bulb.
- Insert syringe into side of mouth, avoiding center of the mouth.
- Suction mouth first, then one nostril, then second nostril.

Ⓝ *NCLEX® Connection: Health Promotion and Maintenance, Ante/Intra/Postpartum and Newborn Care*

CHAPTER 16

Complications of the Newborn

Management of newborn complications includes data collection, identifying risk factors, and collaborative care. It is essential to immediately identify complications and implement appropriate interventions. Ongoing emotional support to the client and significant other is also part of the nursing care.

Complications include neonatal substance withdrawal, hypoglycemia, respiratory distress syndrome (RDS)/asphyxia/meconium aspiration, preterm newborn, small for gestational age newborn, large for gestational age (LGA)/ macrosomic newborn, postmature newborn, newborn infection/sepsis (sepsis neonatorum), and hyperbilirubinemia.

Neonatal substance withdrawal

Maternal substance use during pregnancy consists of any use of alcohol or drugs. Intrauterine drug exposure can cause anomalies, neurobehavioral changes, and evidence of withdrawal in the newborn. These changes depend on the specific drug or combination of drugs used; dosage; route of administration; metabolism and excretion by the mother and fetus; and timing and length of drug exposure.

- Substance withdrawal in the newborn occurs when the mother uses drugs that have addictive properties during pregnancy. This includes illegal drugs, alcohol, tobacco, and prescription medications.
- Fetal alcohol syndrome (FAS) results from chronic or periodic intake of alcohol during pregnancy. Alcohol is considered teratogenic, so daily intake of alcohol increases the risk of FAS. Newborns who have FAS are at risk for congenital physical defects and long-term complications.

LONG-TERM COMPLICATIONS
- Feeding problems
- Central nervous system (CNS) dysfunction (cognitive impairment, cerebral palsy)
- Attention deficit disorder
- Language abnormalities
- Microcephaly
- Delayed growth and development
- Poor maternal-newborn bonding

DATA COLLECTION

RISK FACTORS
- Maternal substance use prior to knowing she is pregnant
- Maternal substance use during pregnancy

EXPECTED FINDINGS

Monitor the newborn for abstinence syndrome (withdrawal) and increased wakefulness using the neonatal abstinence scoring system. Observe the newborn for the following.
- **CNS:** High-pitched, shrill cry; incessant crying; irritability; tremors; hyperactivity with an increased Moro reflex; increased deep-tendon reflexes; increased muscle tone; disturbed sleep pattern; hypertonicity; convulsions
- **Metabolic, vasomotor, respiratory:** Nasal congestion with flaring, frequent yawning, skin mottling, retractions, apnea, tachypnea greater than 60/min, sweating, temperature greater than 37.2° C (99° F)
- **Gastrointestinal:** Poor feeding; regurgitation (projectile vomiting); diarrhea; excessive, uncoordinated, constant sucking

OPIATE WITHDRAWAL: Manifestations of neonatal abstinence syndrome

HEROIN WITHDRAWAL
- Low birth weight
- Small for gestational age (SGA)
- Manifestations of neonatal abstinence syndrome
- Increased risk of sudden infant death syndrome (SIDS)

METHADONE WITHDRAWAL
- Manifestations of neonatal abstinence syndrome
- Increased incidence of seizures
- Higher birth weights (compared to heroin exposure)

MARIJUANA WITHDRAWAL
- Preterm birth, meconium staining
- Long-term effects (deficits in attention, cognition, memory, and motor skills)

AMPHETAMINE WITHDRAWAL: Preterm or SGA, drowsiness, jitteriness, sleep pattern disturbances, respiratory distress, frequent infections, poor weight gain, emotional disturbances, delayed growth and development

ALCOHOL WITHDRAWAL: Jitteriness, irritability, increased tone and reflex responses, seizures

FETAL ALCOHOL SYNDROME
- Facial anomalies: small eyes, flat midface, smooth philtrum, thin upper lip, eyes with wide-spaced appearance, epicanthal folds, strabismus, ptosis, poor suck, small teeth, cleft lip or palate
- Deafness
- Abnormal palmar creases, irregular hair
- Many vital organ anomalies (heart defects, including atrial and ventricular septal defects, tetralogy of Fallot, patent ductus arteriosus)
- Developmental delays and neurologic abnormalities
- Prenatal and postnatal growth delays
- Sleep disturbances

TOBACCO: Prematurity; low birth weight; increased risk for SIDS, bronchitis, pneumonia, and developmental delays

LABORATORY TESTS

Blood tests should be done to differentiate between neonatal drug withdrawal and CNS disorders.
- CBC
- Blood glucose
- Electrolyte imbalance
- Thyroid-stimulating hormone, thyroxine, triiodothyronine
- Drug screen of urine or meconium to reveal the substance used by the mother
- Hair analysis

DIAGNOSTIC PROCEDURES

Chest x-ray for FAS to rule out congenital heart defects

PATIENT-CENTERED CARE

NURSING CARE

Nursing care for maternal substance use and neonatal effects or withdrawal include the following in addition to normal newborn care.
- Observe the newborn for manifestations of withdrawal using the neonatal abstinence scoring system.
- Monitor the newborn's ability to feed and digest intake. Offer small frequent feedings of high-calorie formula; can require gavage feedings.
- Elevate the newborn's head during and following feedings, and burp the newborn to reduce vomiting and aspiration. Qs
- Swaddle the newborn with legs flexed to reduce self-stimulation and protect the skin from abrasions. QEBP
- Offer nonnutritive sucking.
- Monitor the newborn's fluids and electrolytes with skin turgor, mucous membranes, fontanels, daily weights, and I&O.
- Reduce environmental stimuli (decrease lights and noise).
- Cluster care to minimize stimulation.
- Monitor the newborn's blood glucose level closely per facility protocol.
- Maintain skin-to-skin contact to treat hypothermia.
- Try various nipples to compensate for a poor suck reflex.
- Have suction available to reduce the risk for aspiration.
- For newborns who are withdrawing from cocaine, avoid eye contact and use vertical rocking.
- Prevent infection.
- Provide data to child protective services.
- Recognize need for lactation services to evaluate whether breastfeeding is desired or contraindicated to avoid passing narcotics in breast milk. Methadone is not contraindicated during breastfeeding. QTC

MEDICATIONS

Based on the severity of withdrawal manifestations

Morphine sulfate: Opioid

Phenobarbital: Anticonvulsant

INTENDED EFFECT: Decrease CNS irritability and control seizures for newborns who have alcohol or opioid withdrawal.

NURSING ACTIONS
- Check IV site frequently (phenobarbital).
- Check for any medication incompatibilities.

CLIENT EDUCATION
- Participate in referral of the mother to a drug or alcohol treatment center.
- Discuss the importance of SIDS prevention activities due to the increased rate in newborns of mothers who used methadone.

Hypoglycemia

The newborn's source of glucose stops when the umbilical cord is clamped. A healthy term newborn's blood glucose level can drop to 30 mg/dL the first 1 to 2 hr following birth. If newborns have other physiological stress, they can experience hypoglycemia due to inadequate gluconeogenesis or increased use of glycogen stores.

- Hypoglycemia is a serum glucose level less than 40 mg/dl. Glucose levels should be measured in newborns who have risk factors or manifestations of hypoglycemia.
- Untreated hypoglycemia can result in seizures, brain damage, or death.

DATA COLLECTION

RISK FACTORS

- Maternal diabetes mellitus
- Preterm infant
- LGA or SGA
- Stress at birth (cold stress, asphyxia)

EXPECTED FINDINGS

PHYSICAL FINDINGS
- Poor feeding
- Jitteriness/tremors
- Hypothermia
- Diaphoresis
- Weak cry
- Lethargy
- Flaccid muscle tone
- Seizures/coma
- Irregular respirations
- Cyanosis
- Apnea

LABORATORY TESTS

Blood glucose levels less than 45 mg/dL should be followed up with a serum glucose level.

PATIENT-CENTERED CARE

NURSING CARE

- Obtain blood by heel stick for glucose monitoring.
- An asymptomatic at-risk newborn who has a blood glucose 25 mg/dL in the first 4 hr, or less than 35 mg/dL from 4 hr to 24 hr of age, should be offered oral feedings to increase level to greater than 45 mg/dL.
- Provide frequent oral or gavage feedings or continuous parenteral nutrition early after birth to treat hypoglycemia.
- Monitor IV if the newborn is unable to feed orally.

Respiratory distress syndrome, asphyxia, meconium aspiration

- RDS occurs as a result of surfactant deficiency in the lungs and is characterized by poor gas exchange and ventilatory failure.
- Surfactant is a phospholipid that assists in alveoli expansion. Surfactant keeps alveoli from collapsing and allows gas exchange to occur.
- Atelectasis (collapsing of a portion of lung) increases the work of breathing. As a result, respiratory acidosis and hypoxemia can develop.
- Birth weight alone is not an indicator of fetal lung maturity.
- Complications from RDS are related to oxygen therapy and mechanical ventilation.
  - Pneumothorax
  - Retinopathy of prematurity
  - Bronchopulmonary dysplasia
  - Infection
  - Intraventricular hemorrhage

DATA COLLECTION

RISK FACTORS

- Preterm gestation
- Perinatal asphyxia (meconium staining, cord prolapse, nuchal cord)
- Maternal diabetes mellitus
- Premature rupture of membranes
- Maternal use of barbiturates or narcotics close to birth
- Maternal hypotension
- Cesarean birth without labor
- Hydrops fetalis (massive edema of the fetus caused by hyperbilirubinemia)
- Maternal bleeding during the third trimester
- Hypovolemia
- Genetics: male sex, Caucasian descent

EXPECTED FINDINGS

PHYSICAL FINDINGS
- Tachypnea (respiratory rate greater than 60/min)
- Nasal flaring
- Expiratory grunting
- Retractions
- Labored breathing with prolonged expiration
- Fine crackles on auscultation
- Cyanosis
- Unresponsiveness, flaccidity, and apnea with decreased breath sounds (manifestations of worsened RDS)

LABORATORY TESTS

- ABGs
- Complete blood count with differential
- Culture and sensitivity of the blood, urine, and cerebrospinal fluid
- Blood glucose

DIAGNOSTIC PROCEDURES

Chest x-ray

PATIENT-CENTERED CARE

NURSING CARE

- Suction the newborn's mouth, trachea, and nose as needed.
- Maintain thermoregulation.
- Provide mouth and skin care.
- Correct metabolic acidosis by administering sodium bicarbonate.
- Maintain adequate oxygenation, prevent lactic acidosis, and avoid the toxic effects of oxygen.
- Monitor pulse oximetry.
- Monitor parenteral nutrition.
- Monitor laboratory results, I&O, and weight to evaluate hydration status.
- Decrease stimuli.

Preterm newborn

- A preterm newborn's birth occurs after 20 weeks and before completion of 37 weeks of gestation.
- A late preterm newborn's birth occurs from 34 to 36 weeks of gestation.
- An early term newborn's birth occurs from 37 to 38⁶/₇ weeks of gestation.
- Preterm newborns are at risk for complications due to immature organ systems. The degree of complications depends on gestational age. Risk for complications decreases the closer the newborn is to 40 weeks of gestation.
  - Goals include meeting the newborn's growth and development needs, and anticipating and managing associated complications such as RDS and sepsis.
  - The main priority in treating newborns who are preterm is supporting the cardiac and respiratory systems as needed. Most newborns who are preterm are cared for in a neonatal intensive care unit (NICU).

DATA COLLECTION

EXPECTED FINDINGS

PHYSICAL FINDINGS

- Ballard assessment showing a physical and neurological assessment totaling less than 37 weeks of gestation
- Periodic breathing consisting of 5- to 10-second respiratory pauses, followed by 10- to 15-second compensatory rapid respirations
- Manifestations of increased respiratory effort or respiratory distress (nasal flaring or retractions of the chest wall during inspirations, expiratory grunting, tachypnea)
- Apnea: pause in respirations 20 seconds or longer
- Low birth weight
- Minimal subcutaneous fat deposits
- Head that is large in comparison with the body
- Small fontanels
- Wrinkled features with abundance of lanugo covering back, forearms, forehead, and sides of face
- Few or no creases on soles of feet
- Skull and rib cage that feel soft
- Eyes closed if newborn is born at 22 to 24 weeks of gestation
- Weak grasp reflex
- Inability to coordinate suck and swallow; weak or absent gag, suck, and cough reflex; weak swallow
- Hypotonic muscles, decreased level of activity, and a weak cry for more than 24 hr
- Lethargy, tachycardia, poor weight gain

Small for gestational age newborn

- SGA describes a newborn whose birth weight is at or below the 10th percentile and who has intrauterine growth restriction.
- Common complications are perinatal asphyxia, meconium aspiration, hypoglycemia, polycythemia, and instability of body temperature.

DATA COLLECTION

RISK FACTORS

- Congenital or chromosomal anomalies
- Maternal infections, disease, or malnutrition
- Gestational hypertension or diabetes
- Maternal smoking, drug, or alcohol use
- Placental factors (small placenta, placenta previa, decreased placental perfusion)
- Fetal congenital infections such as rubella or toxoplasmosis

EXPECTED FINDINGS

PHYSICAL FINDINGS
- Weight less than 10th percentile
- Normal skull, but reduced body dimensions
- Hair is sparse on scalp
- Wide skull sutures from inadequate bone growth
- Dry, loose skin
- Decreased subcutaneous fat
- Decreased muscle mass, particularly over cheeks and buttocks
- Thin, dry, yellow, dull umbilical cord (rather than gray, glistening, moist)
- Sunken abdomen rather than well-rounded

COMPLICATIONS
- Respiratory distress and hypoxia
- Meconium aspiration
- Hypoglycemia
- Temperature instability

LABORATORY TESTS

- Blood glucose for hypoglycemia
- CBC commonly shows polycythemia resulting from fetal hypoxia and intrauterine stress.
- ABGs may be prescribed due to chronic hypoxia in utero due to placental insufficiency.

DIAGNOSTIC PROCEDURES

Chest x-ray to rule out meconium aspiration syndrome

PATIENT-CENTERED CARE

NURSING CARE

- Support respiratory efforts. Suction the newborn as necessary to maintain an open airway. Qs
- Provide a neutral thermal environment for the newborn (isolette or radiant heat warmer) to prevent cold stress.
- Initiate early feedings. (The newborn will require more frequent feedings.)
- Maintain adequate hydration.
- Conserve the newborn's energy.
- Prevent skin breakdown.
- Protect the newborn from infection.

CLIENT EDUCATION

Provide support to the newborn's parents and extended family, and encourage them to participate in caring for the newborn. Anticipate home care needs. Qpcc

Large for gestational age (macrosomic) newborn

- LGA occurs in newborns who are above the 90th percentile or weigh more than 4,000 g (8 lb, 12.8 oz). Macrosomia is used to described the large body size.
- Newborns who are LGA can be preterm, postmature, or full-term.
- Newborns who are macrosomic are at risk for birth injuries (shoulder dystocia from clavicle fracture or a cesarean birth, asphyxia, hypoglycemia, polycythemia and Erb-Duchenne paralysis due to birth trauma).

DATA COLLECTION

RISK FACTORS

- Newborns who are postmature
- Maternal diabetes mellitus during pregnancy (high glucose levels stimulate continued insulin production by the fetus)
- Fetal cardiovascular disorder of transposition of the great vessels
- Genetic factors
- Maternal obesity
- Multiparity

EXPECTED FINDINGS

PHYSICAL FINDINGS
- Weight greater than 90th percentile (4,000 g)
- Large head
- Plump and full-faced (Cushingoid appearance) from increased subcutaneous fat
- Sluggishness, hypotonic muscles, and hypoactivity

COMPLICATIONS
- Manifestations of hypoxia (tachypnea, retractions, cyanosis, nasal flaring, grunting)
- Birth trauma (fractures, shoulder dystocia, intracranial hemorrhage, CNS injury)
- Hypoglycemia
- Respiratory distress from immature lungs or meconium aspiration
- Findings of increased intracranial pressure (dilated pupils, vomiting, bulging fontanels, high-pitched cry)

LABORATORY TESTS

- Blood glucose levels to monitor closely for hypoglycemia
- ABGs may be prescribed due to chronic hypoxia in utero secondary to placental insufficiency.
- CBC shows polycythemia (Hct greater than 65%) from in utero hypoxia.
- Hyperbilirubinemia resulting from polycythemia as excessive RBCs break down after birth.
- Hypocalcemia can result in response to a long and difficult birth.

PATIENT-CENTERED CARE

NURSING CARE

- Obtain early and frequent heel sticks (blood glucose testing).
- Initiate early feedings or monitor IV therapy to maintain glucose levels within the expected reference range.
- Provide thermoregulation with an isolette.
- Identify and treat any birth injuries.

Postmature (postterm) infant

- A newborn who is postmature is born after the completion of 42 weeks of gestation. Postmaturity of the infant can be associated with either of the following.
  - **Dysmaturity from placental degeneration and uteroplacental insufficiency** (placenta no longer functions effectively after 40 weeks) resulting in chronic fetal hypoxia and fetal distress in utero. The fetal response is polycythemia, meconium aspiration, or neonatal respiratory problems. Perinatal mortality is higher when a postmature placenta fails to meet increased oxygen demands of the fetus during labor.
  - **Continued growth of the fetus in utero** because the placenta continues to function effectively and the newborn becomes LGA at birth. This leads to a difficult delivery and cephalopelvic disproportion, as well as high insulin reserves and insufficient glucose reserves at birth. The neonatal response can be birth trauma, perinatal asphyxia, clavicle fracture, seizures, hypoglycemia, or temperature instability (cold stress).
- A newborn who is postmature can be SGA or LGA depending on how well the placenta functions during the last weeks of pregnancy.
- Newborns who are postmature have an increased risk for aspirating the meconium passed by the fetus in utero.
- Persistent pulmonary hypertension (persistent fetal circulation) can result from meconium aspiration. There is an interference in the transition from fetal to neonatal circulation. The ductus arteriosus (connecting the main pulmonary artery and the aorta) and foramen ovale (shunt between the right and left atria) remain open, and fetal pathways of blood flow continue.

DATA COLLECTION

RISK FACTORS

In most cases, the cause of a pregnancy that extends beyond 40 weeks of gestation is unknown, but there is a higher incidence in first pregnancies and in clients who have had a previous postmature pregnancy.

EXPECTED FINDINGS

PHYSICAL FINDINGS
- Wasted appearance
- Thin with loose skin, having lost some of the subcutaneous fat
- Skin that is peeling, cracked, dry; leathery from decreased protection of vernix and amniotic fluid
- Long, thin body
- Meconium staining of fingernails and umbilical cord
- Long hair and nails
- Alertness similar to a 2-week-old newborn
- Difficulty establishing respirations secondary to meconium aspiration
- Hypoglycemia due to insufficient stores of glycogen
- Findings of cold stress
- Neurological manifestations that become apparent with the development of fine motor skills
- Macrosomia

LABORATORY TESTS

- Blood glucose level to monitor for hypoglycemia
- ABGs secondary to chronic hypoxia in utero due to placental insufficiency
- CBC can show polycythemia from decreased oxygenation in utero
- Hct elevated from polycythemia and dehydration

DIAGNOSTIC PROCEDURES

Chest x-ray to rule out meconium aspiration syndrome

PATIENT-CENTERED CARE

NURSING CARE

- Monitor vital signs.
- Monitor IV fluids.
- Moisturize the skin with a petrolatum-based ointment.
- Administer oxygen.
- Assist with/or monitor exchange transfusion if hematocrit is high.
- Provide thermoregulation in an isolette to avoid cold stress.
- Provide early feedings to avoid hypoglycemia.
- Identify and treat any birth injuries.

THERAPEUTIC PROCEDURES

Cesarean birth

Newborn infection, sepsis neonatorum

- Infection can be contracted by the newborn before, during, or after delivery. Newborns are more susceptible to micro-organisms due to their limited immunity and inability to localize infection. The infection can spread rapidly into the bloodstream.
- Newborn sepsis is the presence of micro-organisms or their toxins in the blood or tissues of the newborn during the first month after birth. Manifestations are subtle and can resemble other diseases; the nurse often notices them during routine care of the newborn.
- Organisms frequently responsible for newborn infections include *Staphylococcus aureus*, *Staphylococcus epidermidis*, *Escherichia coli*, *Haemophilus influenzae*, and Group B streptococcus beta-hemolytic.
- Prevention of infection and newborn sepsis starts perinatally with maternal screening for infections, prophylactic interventions, and the use of sterile and aseptic techniques during delivery. Prophylactic antibiotic treatment of the eyes of all newborns and appropriate umbilical cord care also help to prevent newborn infection and sepsis. Q͟EBP

DATA COLLECTION

RISK FACTORS

- Premature rupture of membranes
- Prolonged labor
- Toxoplasmosis, rubella, cytomegalovirus, and herpes (TORCH)
- Chorioamnionitis
- Preterm birth
- Low birth weight
- Maternal substance use
- Maternal urinary tract infection
- Meconium aspiration

EXPECTED FINDINGS

PHYSICAL FINDINGS

- Temperature instability
- Suspicious drainage (eyes, umbilical stump)
- Poor feeding pattern, such as weak suck or decreased intake
- Vomiting, diarrhea
- Hypoglycemia, hyperglycemia
- Abdominal distention
- Apnea, retractions, grunting, nasal flaring
- Decreased oxygen saturation
- Color changes (pallor, jaundice, petechiae)
- Tachycardia or bradycardia
- Tachypnea
- Low blood pressure
- Irritability, seizure activity
- Poor muscle tone, lethargy

LABORATORY TESTS

- CBC with differential, C-reactive protein
- Blood, urine, and cerebrospinal fluid cultures and sensitivities
- Chemical profile shows a fluid and electrolyte imbalance.

PATIENT-CENTERED CARE

NURSING CARE

- Determine infection risks. (Review maternal health record.)
- Monitor for findings of opportunistic infection.
- Monitor vital signs continuously.
- Monitor I&O and daily weight.
- Monitor fluid and electrolyte status.
- Monitor the newborn's visitors for infection.
- Obtain specimens (blood, urine, stool) to assist in identifying the causative organism.
- Maintain IV therapy to administer electrolyte replacements, fluids, and medications
- Implement isolation precautions as indicated.
- Administer medications (antibiotics, antivirals, antifungals).
- Maintain respiratory support as needed.
- Monitor IV site for evidence of infection.
- Provide newborn care to maintain temperature.
- Clean and sterilize all equipment to be used.
- Provide emotional support to the family.

CLIENT EDUCATION

DISCHARGE INSTRUCTIONS

- Provide the family with education about infection control.
  - Use clean bottles and nipples for each feeding.
  - Discard any unused formula.
  - Supervise hand hygiene.
- Promote adequate rest for newborn, and decrease physical stimulation.

Hyperbilirubinemia

Hyperbilirubinemia is an elevation of serum bilirubin levels resulting in jaundice. Jaundice normally appears on the head (especially the sclera and mucous membranes), and then progresses down the thorax, abdomen, and extremities.

Jaundice can be physiologic or pathologic.

- **Physiologic jaundice** is considered benign (resulting from normal newborn physiology of increased bilirubin production due to the shortened lifespan and breakdown of fetal RBCs and liver immaturity). The newborn who has physiological jaundice exhibits an increase in unconjugated bilirubin levels 72 to 120 hr after birth, with a rapid decline to 3 mg/dL 5 to 10 days after birth.
- **Pathologic jaundice** is a result of an underlying disease. Pathologic jaundice appears before 24 hr of age or is persistent after day 14. In the term newborn, bilirubin levels increase more than 0.5 mg/dL/hr, peaks at greater than 12.9 mg/dL, or is associated with anemia and hepatosplenomegaly. Pathologic jaundice is usually caused by a blood group incompatibility or an infection, but can be the result of RBC disorders.

Acute bilirubin encephalopathy is when the bilirubin is deposited in the brain. This occurs once all of the binding sites for the bilirubin are used within the body, resulting in necrosis of neurons. Bilirubin levels greater than 25 mg/dL place the newborn at risk. This can result in permanent damage (dystonia, athetosis, upward gaze, hearing loss, cognitive impairments).

Kernicterus is an irreversible, chronic result of bilirubin toxicity. The newborn demonstrates many of the manifestations of bilirubin encephalopathy (hypotonia, severe cognitive impairments, spastic quadriplegia).

DATA COLLECTION

RISK FACTORS

- Increased RBC production or breakdown
- Rh or ABO incompatibility
- Decreased liver function
- Maternal ingestion of diazepam, salicylates, or sulfonamides close to birth
- Maternal diabetes
- Oxytocin during labor
- Neonatal hyperthyroidism
- Ecchymosis or hemangioma
- Prematurity

EXPECTED FINDINGS

PHYSICAL FINDINGS

- Yellowish tint to skin, sclera, and mucous membranes
- Jaundice
  - To verify jaundice, press the newborn's skin on the cheek or abdomen lightly with one finger.
  - Lift the finger to release pressure, and observe the newborn's skin color for yellowish tint on the blanched skin.
- Hypoxia, hypothermia, hypoglycemia, and metabolic acidosis can occur as a result of hyperbilirubinemia and can increase the risk of brain damage.

LABORATORY TESTS

- An elevated serum bilirubin level can occur (direct and indirect bilirubin). Monitor the newborn's bilirubin levels every 4 hr until the level returns to normal. Qs
- Identify maternal and newborn blood type to determine whether there is ABO incompatibility. This occurs if the newborn has blood type A or B, and the mother is type O.
- Review Hgb and Hct.
- A direct Coombs' test reveals the presence of antibody-coated (sensitized) Rh-positive RBCs in the newborn.
- Check electrolyte levels for dehydration from phototherapy.

DIAGNOSTIC PROCEDURES

Transcutaneous bilirubin level is a noninvasive method to measure bilirubin level.

PATIENT-CENTERED CARE

NURSING CARE

- Observe the skin and mucous membranes for jaundice. Document the time of jaundice onset.
- Monitor vital signs.
- Provide care for newborns receiving phototherapy.
  - Maintain an eye mask over the newborn's eyes for protection of corneas and retinas.
  - Keep the newborn undressed. For a male newborn, a surgical mask should be placed (like a bikini) over the genitalia to prevent possible testicular damage from heat and light waves. Be sure to remove the metal strip from the mask to prevent burning. QEBP
  - Avoid applying lotions or ointments to the skin because they absorb heat and can cause burns.
  - Remove the newborn from phototherapy every 4 hr and unmask the newborn's eyes, checking for inflammation or injury.
  - Reposition the newborn every 2 hr to expose all of the body surfaces to the phototherapy lights and prevent pressure sores.
  - Check the lamp energy with a photometer per facility protocol.
  - Turn off the phototherapy lights before drawing blood for testing.

- Observe the newborn for effects of phototherapy.
  - Bronze discoloration (not a serious complication)
  - Maculopapular skin rash (not a serious complication)
  - Development of pressure areas
  - Dehydration (poor skin turgor, dry mucous membranes, decreased urinary output)
  - Elevated temperature
- Encourage the parents to hold and interact with the newborn when phototherapy lights are off.
- Monitor elimination and daily weights, watching for evidence of dehydration.
- Check the newborn's axillary temperature every 4 hr during phototherapy because temperature can become elevated.
- Feed the newborn early and frequently, every 3 to 4 hr. This will promote bilirubin excretion in the stools.
- Encourage continued breastfeeding of the newborn. Supplementation with formula may be prescribed.
- Maintain adequate fluid intake to prevent dehydration.
- Reassure the parents that most newborns experience some degree of jaundice.
- Explain that the newborn's stool contains some bile that will be loose and green.

THERAPEUTIC PROCEDURES

Phototherapy: The newborn's bilirubin should start to decrease within 4 to 6 hr after starting treatment.

CLIENT EDUCATION

DISCHARGE INSTRUCTIONS
- Educate parents regarding the newborn's plan of care.
- Infants who have low to moderate risk of hyperbilirubinemia should receive follow-up care within 2 days. Infants at higher risk should be seen within 24 hr.

PRACTICE Active Learning Scenario

A nurse educator is reviewing hyperbilirubinemia with a newly hired nurse. What should the nurse educator include in this review? Use the ATI Active Learning Template: System Disorder to complete this item.

ALTERATION IN HEALTH (DIAGNOSIS): Describe the difference between physiologic and pathologic jaundice, acute bilirubin encephalopathy, and kernicterus.

DIAGNOSTIC PROCEDURES: Describe the procedure that can be used to verify the presence of jaundice.

NURSING CARE: Describe care of the newborn receiving phototherapy.

Application Exercises

1. A nurse is assisting with the care of a client who is at 42 weeks gestation and in labor. The client asks the nurse what should she expect because her baby is postmature. Which of the following statements should the nurse make?

   A. "Your baby will have excess body fat."

   B. "Your baby will have flat areola without breast buds."

   C. "Your baby's heels will easily move to his ears."

   D. "Your baby's skin will have a leathery appearance."

2. A nurse is caring for an infant who has a high bilirubin level and is receiving phototherapy. Which of the following is the priority finding in the newborn?

   A. Conjunctivitis

   B. Bronze skin discoloration

   C. Sunken fontanels

   D. Maculopapular skin rash

3. A nurse is assisting with data collection of a newborn who was born at 32 weeks of gestation. The newborn's birth weight is 1,100 g. Which of the following findings should the nurse expect? (Select all that apply.)

   A. Lanugo

   B. Long nails

   C. Weak grasp reflex

   D. Translucent skin

   E. Plump face

4. A nurse is assisting with data collection of a postterm newborn. Which of the following findings should the nurse expect? (Select all that apply.)

   A. Thin with loose skin

   B. Increased amount of vernix

   C. Increased amount of lanugo

   D. Meconium staining of umbilical cord

   E. Long finger nails

5. A nurse is discussing neonatal abstinence syndrome with a newly licensed nurse. Which of the following statements by the newly licensed nurse indicate understanding?

   A. "The newborn will have decreased muscle tone."

   B. "The newborn will have a continuous high-pitched cry."

   C. "The newborn will sleep for 2 to 3 hours after a feeding."

   D. "The newborn will have mild tremors when disturbed."

Application Exercises Key

1. A. Excess body fat is seen in a newborn who is macrosomic.

   B. Flat areolas without breast buds are seen in a newborn who is preterm.

   C. Heels that are movable fully to the ears are seen in newborn who is preterm.

   D. **CORRECT:** Leathery, cracked, and wrinkled skin is seen in a newborn who is postmature due to placental insufficiency.

   Ⓝ *NCLEX® Connection: Physiological Adaptation, Alterations in Body Systems*

2. A. Conjunctivitis is a minor complication of phototherapy. Another finding is the priority.

   B. Bronze skin discoloration is a minor complication of phototherapy. Another finding is the priority.

   C. **CORRECT:** The greatest risk to this client is injury from dehydration. Sunken fontanels is the priority finding.

   D. Maculopapular skin rash is a minor complication of phototherapy. Another finding is the priority.

   Ⓝ *NCLEX® Connection: Health Promotion and Maintenance, Health Promotion/Disease Prevention*

3. A. **CORRECT:** Characteristics of a preterm newborn include the presence of abundant lanugo.

   B. Long nails are a finding in a newborn who is postmature.

   C. **CORRECT:** A weak grasp reflex is characteristic of a preterm newborn.

   D. **CORRECT:** Skin that is thin, smooth, shiny, and translucent is a finding in a preterm newborn.

   E. A plump face would be observed in a newborn who is macrosomic.

   Ⓝ *NCLEX® Connection: Health Promotion and Maintenance, Data Collection Techniques*

4. A. **CORRECT:** Wasted appearance, thin with loose skin, and having lost some of the subcutaneous fat are characteristics of postterm newborns

   B. Characteristics of a preterm newborn include an abundant amount of vernix.

   C. Characteristics of a preterm newborn include the presence of abundant lanugo.

   D. **CORRECT:** Meconium staining of fingernails and umbilical cord are manifestations of postterm newborns.

   E. **CORRECT:** Long nails and hair are findings in a newborn who is postterm.

   Ⓝ *NCLEX® Connection: Health Promotion and Maintenance, Data Collection Techniques*

5. A. Increased muscle tone is seen in a newborn who has neonatal abstinence syndrome.

   B. **CORRECT:** A continuous high-pitched cry is often an indication of CNS disturbances in a newborn who has neonatal abstinence syndrome.

   C. A newborn who has neonatal abstinence syndrome can have sleep pattern disturbances and would have difficulty sleeping for 2 to 3 hr after feeding.

   D. A newborn who has neonatal abstinence syndrome often has moderate to severe tremors when undisturbed. Most newborns exhibit mild tremors when disturbed.

   Ⓝ *NCLEX® Connection: Physiological Adaptation, Alterations in Body Systems*

PRACTICE Answer

Using the ATI Active Learning Template: System Disorder

ALTERATION IN HEALTH (DIAGNOSIS)
- Physiologic jaundice is considered benign (resulting from normal newborn physiology of increased bilirubin production due to the shortened lifespan and breakdown of fetal RBCs and liver immaturity). The newborn who has physiological jaundice exhibits an increase in unconjugated bilirubin levels 72 to 120 hr after birth, with a rapid decline to 3 mg/dL 5 to 10 days after birth.
- Pathologic jaundice is a result of an underlying disease. Pathologic jaundice appears before 24 hr of age or is persistent after day 14. In the term newborn, bilirubin levels increase more than 0.5 mg/dL/hr, peak at greater than 12.9 mg/dL, or are associated with anemia and hepatosplenomegaly. Pathologic jaundice is usually caused by a blood group incompatibility or an infection, but can be the result of RBC disorders.
- Acute bilirubin encephalopathy is when the bilirubin is deposited in the brain. This occurs once all of the binding sites for the bilirubin are used within the body, resulting in necrosis of neurons. Bilirubin greater than 25 mg/dL places the newborn at risk for permanent damage, including dystonia, athetosis, upward gaze, hearing loss, and cognitive impairments.
- Kernicterus is an irreversible, chronic result of bilirubin toxicity. The newborn demonstrates many of the same manifestations of bilirubin encephalopathy (hypotonia, severe cognitive impairments, spastic quadriplegia).

DIAGNOSTIC PROCEDURES: Press the newborn's skin on the cheek or abdomen lightly with one finger. Then release pressure, and observe for a yellowish tint to the skin as the skin is blanched.

NURSING CARE
- Maintain an eye mask over the newborn's eyes.
- Keep the newborn undressed. Place a mask (like a bikini) over the genitalia of a male newborn.
- Remove the newborn from phototherapy every 4 hr, and unmask the eyes.
- Reposition the newborn every 2 hr to expose all body surfaces to the phototherapy lights and prevent pressure sores.
- Check the lamp energy with a photometer following facility protocol.
- Turn off the phototherapy lights before drawing blood for testing.

Ⓝ *NCLEX® Connection: Physiological Adaptation, Alterations in Body Systems*

UNIT 4 NEWBORN NURSING CARE
Baby-Friendly Care

Bonding and integration of a newborn into the family structure should start during pregnancy, and continue into the fourth stage of labor and throughout hospitalization.

Observation of bonding and integration of a newborn into the family structure requires that a nurse understand the expected postpartum psychological changes the client undergoes in the attainment of the maternal role and recognize deviations. Baby-friendly care can be promoted by delaying nursing procedures during the first hour after birth and through the first attempt of the client to breastfeed to allow for immediate parent-newborn contact.

A client's emotional and physical condition (unwanted pregnancy, adolescent pregnancy, history of depression, difficult pregnancy and birth) and the newborn's physical condition (prematurity, congenital anomalies) can affect the family's bonding process. Culture, age, and socioeconomic level can influence the bonding process. Nurses can recognize actual and potential problems related to the bonding process and work together with other disciplines to ensure adequate care for the parents after discharge. If needed, prior to discharge, the nurse should make referrals to social services or community agencies.

PSYCHOSOCIAL AND MATERNAL ADAPTATION

Psychosocial adaptation and maternal adjustment begin during pregnancy as the client goes through commitment, attachment, and preparation for the birth of the newborn.

- During the first 2 to 6 weeks after birth, the client goes through a period of acquaintance with the newborn, as well as physical restoration. During this time she also focuses on competently caring for the newborn.
- Finally, the act of achieving maternal identity is accomplished around 4 months following birth.
- These stages can overlap, and are variable based on maternal, newborn, and the environmental factors.

PHASES OF MATERNAL ROLE ATTAINMENT

Dependent: taking-in phase
- First 24 to 48 hr
- Focus on meeting personal needs
- Rely on others for assistance
- Excited, talkative
- Need to review birth experience with others

Dependent–independent: taking-hold phase
- Begins on day 2 or 3
- Lasts 10 days to several weeks
- Focus on baby care and improving caregiving competency
- Want to take charge but need acceptance from others
- Want to learn and practice
- Dealing with physical and emotional discomforts
- Can experience "baby blues"

Interdependent: letting-go phase
- Focus on family as a unit
- Resumption of role (intimate partner, individual)

DATA COLLECTION

Check the client's condition after birth, observe the maternal adaptation process, determine maternal emotional readiness to care for the newborn, and observe how comfortable the client appears in providing newborn care.
- Observe for behaviors that facilitate and indicate mother-newborn bonding.
  - Considers the newborn a family member
  - Holds the newborn face-to-face (en face position), maintaining eye contact
  - Assigns meaning to the newborn's behavior and views this positively
  - Identifies the newborn's unique characteristics and relates them to those of other family members
  - Names the newborn
  - Touches the newborn and maintains close physical proximity
  - Provides physical care for the newborn (feeding, diapering)
  - Responds to the newborn's cries
  - Smiles at, talks to, and sings to the newborn

- Monitor for behaviors that impair and indicate a lack of mother-newborn bonding.
  - Apathy when the newborn cries
  - Disgust when the newborn voids, defecates, or spits up
  - Expresses disappointment in the newborn
  - Turns away from the newborn often
  - Does not seek close physical proximity to the newborn
  - Does not talk about the newborn's unique features
  - Handles the newborn roughly
  - Ignores the newborn entirely
  - Does not include the newborn in the family context
  - Perceives newborn behavior as uncooperative
- Monitor for manifestations of mood swings, conflict about maternal role, or personal insecurity.
  - Feelings of being "down"
  - Feelings of inadequacy
  - Feelings of anxiety related to ineffective breastfeeding
  - Emotional lability with frequent crying
  - Flat affect and being withdrawn
  - Feeling unable to care for the newborn

NURSING ACTIONS

- Facilitate the bonding process by placing the newborn skin-to-skin and face-to-face with the mother immediately after birth.
- Promote rooming-in as a quiet and private environment that enhances the family bonding process.
- Promote early initiation of breastfeeding, and encourage the client to recognize newborn readiness cues. Offer assistance as needed.
- Reinforce that newborn care facilitates bonding as the client's confidence improves.
- Encourage parent bonding with the newborn through cuddling, bathing, feeding, diapering, and inspection.
- Provide frequent praise, support, and reassurance to the mother as she moves toward independence in caring for her newborn and adjusting to her maternal role.
- Encourage parents to express feelings, fears, and anxieties about caring for the newborn.

PATERNAL ADAPTATION

Paternal adaptation takes place as the father develops a parent-newborn bond.
- The father has skin-to-skin contact, holds the newborn, and maintains eye contact with the newborn.
- The father observes the newborn for features similar to his own to validate his claim of the newborn.
- The father talks, sings, and reads to the newborn.

TRANSITION

Paternal transition to fatherhood consists of a predictable four-stage process during the first few weeks of transition.

Expectations and intentions: The father desires to be deeply and emotionally connected with the newborn.

Confronting reality: The father discovers that his expectations might not be met. Commonly expressed emotions include sadness, frustration, and jealousy. He embraces the need to be actively involved in parenting.

Creating the role of the involved father: The father decides to become actively involved in the care of the newborn.

Reaping rewards: Rewards include newborn smiles and a sense of completeness and meaning.

DATA COLLECTION

The nurse can determine if paternal adaptation has occurred by observing for the characteristics of father-newborn bonding.

NURSING ACTIONS

- Reinforce education about newborn care when the father is present, and encourage the father to take a hands-on approach.
- Assist the father in his transition to fatherhood by providing guidance and involving him as a full partner rather than just a helper.
- Encourage couples to verbalize concerns and expectations related to newborn care.

SIBLING ADAPTATION

The addition of a newborn into the family unit affects everyone in the family, including siblings who can experience a temporary separation from parents. Siblings become aware of changes in the parents' behavior because the newborn requires much more of parents' time.

DATA COLLECTION

The nurse can determine if sibling adaptation to the newborn has occurred.
- Observe for positive responses from siblings.
  - Interest and concern for the newborn
  - Increased independence
- Monitor for adverse responses from siblings.
  - Indications of sibling rivalry and jealousy
  - Regression in toileting and sleep habits
  - Aggression toward the newborn
  - Increased attention-seeking behaviors and whining

NURSING ACTIONS

- Take siblings on a tour of the obstetric unit.
- Encourage parents to do the following.
  - Let siblings be among the first to see the newborn.
  - Provide a gift from the newborn to give the siblings.
  - Arrange for another caregiver to spend time with the siblings while the parent is caring for the newborn.
  - Allow older siblings to help provide care for the newborn.
  - Give preschool-aged siblings a doll to care for.

COMPLICATIONS

Impaired parenting can include the following.

- Emotional detachment and inability to care for the newborn, thus placing the newborn at risk for neglect and failure to thrive.
- Failure to bond with the newborn increases the risk of physical and emotional abuse.

NURSING ACTIONS

- Emphasize verbal and nonverbal communication skills between the client, caregivers, and newborn.
- Provide continued monitoring of the client's and caregivers' parenting abilities.
- Encourage continued support of grandparents and other family members.
- Provide home visits and group sessions for discussion regarding newborn care and parenting problems.
- Give the client and caregivers information about social networks that provide a support system where they can seek assistance.
- Involve outreach programs concerned with self–care, parent–child interactions, child injuries, and failure to thrive.
- Notify programs that provide prompt and effective community interventions to prevent more serious problems from occurring.

PRACTICE Active Learning Scenario

A nurse is leading a parenting class on paternal adaptation for pregnant women and their partners. What concepts on paternal adaptation should the nurse include in the presentation? Use ATI Active Learning Template: Basic Concept to complete this item.

RELATED CONTENT: Describe three ways the partner develops a parent-newborn bond.

UNDERLYING PRINCIPLES
- Describe three stages of paternal transition to parenthood.
- Describe three stages of the development of the father-newborn bond.

NURSING INTERVENTIONS: Describe three actions to assist in the father-newborn bonding process.

Application Exercises

1. A nurse notes that the father appears nervous when the mother asks him to help care for the newborn. Which of the following actions should the nurse take to promote father-newborn bonding?

   A. Hand the newborn to the father, and suggest that he change the diaper.

   B. Ask the father why he is so nervous about helping with the newborn.

   C. Tell the father that he will grow accustomed to the newborn.

   D. Reinforce education about newborn care when the father is present.

2. A nurse is caring for a client who is in the early postpartum period and is very excited and talkative. The nurse is having difficulty completing the postpartum data collection. Which of the following actions should the nurse take?

   A. Come back later when the client is less talkative.

   B. Give the client time to express her feelings.

   C. Tell the client she needs to stop talking so data can be collected.

   D. Redirect the client's attention to something other than herself.

3. A nurse is caring for a client who is 1 day postpartum. The nurse is checking for maternal adaptation and bonding with the newborn. For which of the following client behaviors should the nurse intervene? (Select all that apply.)

   A. Demonstrates apathy when the newborn cries

   B. Touches the newborn while maintaining close physical proximity

   C. Views the newborn's behavior as uncooperative during diaper changing

   D. Identifies and relates newborn's characteristics to those of family members

   E. Interprets the newborn's behavior as a meaningful way of expressing needs

4. A nurse is caring for a client who is 2 days postpartum. The client states, "My 4-year old son was toilet trained and now he is frequently wetting himself." Which of the following responses should the nurse make?

   A. "Your son was probably not ready for toilet training and should wear training pants."

   B. "Your son is exhibiting an expected behavior to having a new sibling."

   C. "Your son will need counseling to fix this behavior."

   D. "You should try sending your son to preschool to resolve the behavior."

5. A nurse on a postpartum unit is planning to promote bonding with the family and siblings of a newborn. Which of the following actions should the nurse take?

   A. Encourage the parents to explore the newborn's features.

   B. Limit the amount of time the siblings spend at the hospital.

   C. Suggest to the parents they should place the newborn in the nursery at night for sleeping.

   D. Suggest that the siblings wait until the newborn goes home to hold him.

Application Exercises Key

1. A. It is not helpful to push the father into newborn care activities without first reinforcing education.

   B. This is a nontherapeutic statement and presumes the nurse knows what the father is feeling.

   C. This is a nontherapeutic statement and offers the nurse's opinion.

   D. **CORRECT:** Nursing interventions to promote paternal bonding include reinforcing education about newborn care and encouraging the father to take a hands-on approach.

   Ⓝ NCLEX® Connection: Health Promotion and Maintenance, Ante/Intra/Postpartum and Newborn Care

2. A. The nurse should continue activities while encouraging the client to talk.

   B. **CORRECT:** The nurse should recognize that the client in is the taking-in phase, which begins immediately following birth and lasts a few hours to a couple of days.

   C. It is not necessary for the client to stop talking while the nurse collects data. This response is nontherapeutic.

   D. The client is in the taking-in phase, which includes talking about the birth experience. The client should be encouraged to verbalize her feelings.

   Ⓝ NCLEX® Connection: Health Promotion and Maintenance, Data Collection Techniques

3. A. **CORRECT:** Apathy is a lack of concern or interest in the newborn. This demonstrates impaired maternal-newborn bonding.

   B. Touching the newborn and maintaining close proximity are indications of effective maternal-newborn bonding.

   C. **CORRECT:** A client's view of her newborn as being uncooperative during diaper changing is an indication of impaired maternal-newborn bonding.

   D. Endowing the newborn with family characteristics indicates effective maternal-infant bonding.

   E. Recognizing the newborn's behavior as a meaningful way to express needs is an indication of effective maternal-newborn bonding.

   Ⓝ NCLEX® Connection: Health Promotion and Maintenance, Ante/Intra/Postpartum and Newborn Care

4. A. This is nontherapeutic response by the nurse because it overlooks the child's emotional response to a new family member.

   B. **CORRECT:** The nurse should reassure the mother that this is an expected behavior for a sibling to exhibit. Regression can effect toileting and the sibling's sleep routine. The nurse should also inform the mother that sibling adaptation can include other negative behaviors (seeking attention, frequent complaints, showing hostility toward the baby).

   C. Recommending that the child receive counseling is a nontherapeutic response for a child who is demonstrating an expected sibling response.

   D. Recommending that the child be sent to preschool does not address the parent's concern about a child who is demonstrating regression, which is an expected sibling response.

   Ⓝ NCLEX® Connection: Health Promotion and Maintenance, Developmental Stages and Transitions

5. A. **CORRECT:** The nurse should encourage the parents to explore their newborn, noting the baby's unique features and qualities, to promote parental adaptation.

   B. The nurse should encourage the siblings to visit the hospital and see the newborn as often as they desire to promote family bonding.

   C. The nurse should encourage rooming-in to promote parental bonding and adaptation to the newborn.

   D. The nurse should encourage the parents to allow the siblings to hold the infant at the hospital. This action facilitates sibling acceptance of a new baby.

   Ⓝ NCLEX® Connection: Health Promotion and Maintenance, Ante/Intra/Postpartum and Newborn Care

---

PRACTICE Answer

Using the ATI Active Learning Template: Basic Concept

RELATED CONTENT
- Development of parent-newborn bond
- Touching, holding, skin-to-skin contact, and maintaining eye-to-eye contact
- Recognizing personal features in the newborn, and validating the parent's claim to the newborn
- Talking to, singing to, and verbally interacting with the newborn

UNDERLYING PRINCIPLES
- Stages of paternal transition to parenthood
  - Expectations: Having preconceived ideas about fatherhood
  - Reality: Recognizing expectations might not be met, facing these feelings, and then embracing the need to become actively involved in parenting
  - Transition to mastery: Taking an active role in parenting
- Development of the father-newborn bond
  - Making a commitment and assuming responsibility for parenting
  - Becoming connected and having feelings of attachment to the newborn
  - Modifying lifestyle to make room to care for the newborn

NURSING INTERVENTIONS
- Reinforce education about newborn care when the father is present.
- Encourage the father to take a hands-on role in care when present.
- Provide guidance.
- Involve the father as a full partner, not a helper, in the parenting process.
- Encourage the couple to verbalize concerns and expectations about newborn care.

Ⓝ NCLEX® Connection: Health Promotion and Maintenance, Ante/Intra/Postpartum and Newborn Care

References

Berman, A., Snyder, S., & Frandsen, G. (2016). *Kozier & Erb's fundamentals of nursing: Concepts, process, and practice* (10th ed.). Upper Saddle River, NJ: Prentice-Hall.

Burchum, J. R., & Rosenthal, L. D. (2016). *Lehne's pharmacology for nursing care* (9th ed.). St. Louis, MO: Elsevier.

Centers for Disease Control and Prevention. (2017). *Vaccines and immunizations*. Retrieved from https://www.cdc.gov/vaccines/index.html

Dudek, S. G. (2014). *Nutrition essentials for nursing practice* (7th ed.). Philadelphia: Lippincott Williams & Wilkins.

Grodner, M., Escott-Stump, S., & Dorner, S. (2016). *Nutritional foundations and clinical applications of nutrition: A nursing approach* (6th ed.). St. Louis, MO: Mosby.

Halter, M. J. (2014). *Varcarolis' foundations of psychiatric mental health nursing: A clinical approach* (7th ed.). St. Louis, MO: Saunders.

Hockenberry, M. J., & Wilson, D. (2015) *Wong's nursing care of infants and children* (10th ed.). St. Louis, MO: Mosby.

Immunization Action Coalition. (2017). *Advisory Committee on Immunization Practice*. Retrieved from http://www.immunize.org/acip/

Lowdermilk, D. L., Perry, S. E., Cashion, M. C., & Aldean, K. R. (2016). *Maternity & women's health care* (11th ed.). St. Louis, MO: Elsevier.

Pagana, K. D., & Pagana, T. J. (2014). *Mosby's manual of diagnostic and laboratory tests* (5th ed.). St. Louis, MO: Elsevier.

Pillitteri, A. (2014). *Maternal and child health nursing: Care of the childbearing and childrearing family* (7th ed.). Philadelphia: Lippincott Williams & Wilkins

Potter, P. A., Perry, A. G., Stockert, P., & Hall, A. (2017). *Fundamentals of nursing* (9th ed.). St. Louis, MO: Elsevier

Taketomo, C. K., Hodding, J. H., & Kraus, D. M. (2016). *Lexi-Comp's pediatric & neonatal dosage handbook: A universal resource for clinicians treating pediatric and neonatal patients* (23rd ed.). Hudson, OH: Lexi-Comp.

Vallerand, A.H. & Sanoski, C.A. (2017). *Davis's drug guide for nurses* (15th Ed.). Philadelphia: Elsevier.

STUDENT NAME _____

CONCEPT_____   REVIEW MODULE CHAPTER_____

Related Content

(E.G., DELEGATION, LEVELS OF PREVENTION, ADVANCE DIRECTIVES)

Underlying Principles

Nursing Interventions

WHO? WHEN? WHY? HOW?

ACTIVE LEARNING TEMPLATE: Diagnostic Procedure

STUDENT NAME _____

PROCEDURE NAME _____   REVIEW MODULE CHAPTER_____

Description of Procedure

Indications

CONSIDERATIONS

Nursing Interventions (pre, intra, post)

Interpretation of Findings

Client Education

Potential Complications

Nursing Interventions

ACTIVE LEARNING TEMPLATE: Growth and Development

STUDENT NAME _____

DEVELOPMENTAL STAGE _____   REVIEW MODULE CHAPTER_____

EXPECTED GROWTH AND DEVELOPMENT

Physical Development	Cognitive Development	Psychosocial Development	Age-Appropriate Activities

Health Promotion

Immunizations	Health Screening	Nutrition	Injury Prevention

STUDENT NAME _____

MEDICATION _____ REVIEW MODULE CHAPTER_____

CATEGORY CLASS_____

PURPOSE OF MEDICATION

Expected Pharmacological Action

Therapeutic Use

Complications

Medication Administration

Contraindications/Precautions

Nursing Interventions

Interactions

Client Education

Evaluation of Medication Effectiveness

STUDENT NAME _____

SKILL NAME_____ REVIEW MODULE CHAPTER_____

Description of Skill

Indications

CONSIDERATIONS

Nursing Interventions (pre, intra, post)

Outcomes/Evaluation

Client Education

Potential Complications

Nursing Interventions

System Disorder

STUDENT NAME _____

DISORDER/DISEASE PROCESS _____ REVIEW MODULE CHAPTER_____

Alterations in Health (Diagnosis)	Pathophysiology Related to Client Problem	Health Promotion and Disease Prevention

ASSESSMENT

Risk Factors	Expected Findings

Laboratory Tests	Diagnostic Procedures

SAFETY CONSIDERATIONS

PATIENT-CENTERED CARE

Nursing Care	Medications	Client Education

Therapeutic Procedures		Interprofessional Care

Complications

STUDENT NAME _____

PROCEDURE NAME _____   REVIEW MODULE CHAPTER_____

Description of Procedure

Indications

CONSIDERATIONS

Nursing Interventions (pre, intra, post)

Outcomes/Evaluation

Client Education

Potential Complications

Nursing Interventions